D1521228

PERFORMANCE APPRAISAL FOR PRODUCTIVITY

The Nurse Manager's Handbook

Joan M. Ganong,
R.N., Ph.D., C.M.C.
and
Warren L. Ganong,
C.M.C.

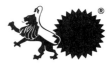

AN ASPEN PUBLICATION ®
Aspen Systems Corporation
Rockville, Maryland
Royal Tunbridge Wells
1984

Library of Congress Cataloging in Publication Data

Ganong, Joan M.
Performance appraisal for productivity.

"An Aspen publication."
Includes bibliographies and index.
1. Nurses—Rating of—Handbooks, manuals, etc. 2. Nursing—
Labor productivity—Handbooks, manuals, etc. 3. Performance
standards—Handbooks, manuals, etc. I. Ganong, Warren L. II.
Title. [DNLM: 1. Efficiency. 2. Nursing, Supervisory.
3. Personnel management. 4. Employee performance appraisal.
WY 30 G198p]
RT85.5.G36   1983   362.1'73'0683   83-15676
ISBN: 0-89443-945-6

Publisher: John Marozsan
Editorial Director: Darlene Como
Executive Managing Editor: Margot Raphael
Editorial Services: Martha Sasser
Printing and Manufacturing: Debbie Collins

Copyright © 1984 by Aspen Systems Corporation

Library of Congress Catalog Card Number: 83-15676
ISBN: 0-89443-945-6

Printed in the United States of America

1   2   3   4   5

Table of Contents

Preface

Performance appraisal. Productivity.

Value-laden, emotionally charged, imprecise concepts? Or welcome, well-understood daily concerns of goal-oriented nurse managers? Perhaps both—among different members of the same organization.

The purpose of this book is to contribute to understanding of the nurse manager's role in performance appraisal for productivity in today's increasingly complex workworld of health care. In addition, guidelines are provided for modernizing outdated performance appraisal techniques and relating these to the initiation of in-house or systemwide career ladders. It is designed for nurse managers in both nursing practice and nursing education settings.

Productivity is a measure of the effective utilization of both capital resources and human resources as related to the organization's mission. Thus, in a nursing department of a health care organization, the nurse manager at each level has accountability and responsibility for carrying out departmental goals and objectives as related to the facility's overall mission. At the practical level, this means using both the technical mode and the human mode (high tech/high touch) in performing the management functions, techniques, and skills. (The use of management terminology here is consistent with the glossary in *Nursing Management* [Ganong & Ganong, 1980].)

Ultimately, of course, it is the performance of every individual that—in the composite—brings about the productivity results, however measured. The ultimate repository of both accountability and responsibility is within each individual. After all, the smallest unit of organization is the individual.

It is the role of the nurse manager to obtain the level of personal and group performance that produces optimal results in the interest of patient care, whatever the available combination of capital and human resources.

This is no small task. It encompasses the whole spectrum of managerial competence, including wise use of performance appraisal. The focus here is on the aspects of performance appraisal that go to the very heart of the employer-employee relationship.

The content is arranged in three groupings. The first three chapters provide a historical overview of performance appraisal and productivity, research findings and existing dilemmas, and organizing for performance appraisal in the context of changing health care concepts. Chapters 4 and 5 present a model for a criteria-based appraisal plan that has been implemented successfully over the years in many hospitals and other health care organizations. Chapters 6 and 7 offer guidance in implementing career ladders that are integrated with the performance appraisal program and present a model for clinical performance appraisal of students of nursing.

At the end of each chapter is a continuing case study titled *For Discussion Purposes* intended to integrate the chapters and stimulate a broader comprehension of the implications of each. Use of these discussions will permit greater understanding of both the process and content of the book's subject matter.

The extensive appendixes include examples of performance appraisal forms, job performance descriptions, career ladder programs, and related materials contributed by a variety of health care organizations, large and small. The examples range from the quite simple to the more complex. Each one is included for a particular reason. One job description, for example, refers to the appropriate standard of the Joint Commission on Accreditation of Hospitals (JCAH), or other standard, as part of every major responsibility listed, as well as coding the level of authority that goes with each responsibility.

Altogether the appendixes provide a major resource representing the creative effort of many nurse managers and other health care personnel across the country. Only a representative few of the forms, etc., available at these institutions are used so as to avoid duplications yet show the range of types and varieties in use.

We hope readers will find this book of continuing value in their quest for managerial competence for the benefit of themselves, their patients, their fellow employees—and, where pertinent, their stockholders.

Joan and Warren Ganong
Chapel Hill, North Carolina

NOTE

Ganong, J.M., & Ganong, W.L. *Nursing management* (2nd. ed.). Rockville, Md.: Aspen Systems Corporation, 1980.

Acknowledgments

We sincerely thank the organizations and managers listed below for permitting inclusion of their materials in the appendixes:

Allen Memorial Hospital, Waterloo, Iowa, Joan I. Headington, Assistant Vice President, Nursing and John C. Omel, Vice President, Employee Services; with credit to Ellen Elsbury, Vice President, Nursing.

Baptist Medical Center at Columbia, Columbia, S.C., Caroline N. Seigler, Vice President.

Charlotte Rehabilitation Hospital, Charlotte, N.C., Kay Rudisill, R.N., Assistant Administrator, Director of Nursing.

Jenkins Methodist Home, Watertown, S.D., Mary Cordell, Director of Nursing Service.

Johnston-Willis Hospital, Richmond, Va., Edna Loving, Director of Nursing.

Loma Linda University Medical Center, Loma Linda, Calif., Job Description Committee, Marilyn Thungquest, Chairman, Nursing Division, and Gertrude Haussler, Vice President.

Mary Greeley Medical Center, Ames, Iowa, Phyllis Crouse, Assistant Administrator, Director of Nursing.

Moses H. Cone Memorial Hospital, Greensboro, N.C., Russell E. Tranbarger, C.N.A.A., Administrator for Nursing.

New England Medical Center, Boston, Mass., Kathleen A. Bower, Associate Chairman, Department of Nursing.

Presbyterian Hospital of Pacific Medical Center, San Francisco, Kenneth Petron, Director, Personnel Service.

St. John's Hospital, Red Wing, Minn., Ruth A. Erickson, Director of Nursing.

St. Mary's Hospital, Milwaukee, Marjorie P. Davis, Assistant Administrator.

Sharon General Hospital, Sharon, Pa., Louise C. Hess, R.N., Vice President, Patient Services; Director of Nursing.

We appreciate just as much the many others whose examples could not be included because of space limitations. Acknowledgment of other valuable source materials is included throughout the text. Tables, figures, and exhibits not credited otherwise are by the authors. Anita Marten, our talented client services manager, has our continuing thanks and affection for her skilled contributions to the preparation of the manuscript while maintaining a sense of order amid impending disasters.

Chapter 1

Performance Appraisal in Perspective

HISTORICAL OVERVIEW

The techniques of performance appraisal in industry generally, and in hospital nursing departments in particular, have received great attention in the last two decades but as recently as the beginning of the 1970s an American Hospital Association booklet on performance appraisal programs concluded, ". . . the failure rate of employee appraisal systems is alarmingly high" (AHA, 1971). Even near the end of that decade another health care author wrote, "The majority of appraisal systems currently in use are neither effective nor valid . . ." (Olmos, 1979).

Yet during this period significant progress was taking place. Some of the developments were stimulated by the Civil Rights Act of 1964 and the later Equal Employment Opportunity Commission (EEOC) guidelines of 1966 and 1970 (DeVries, Morrison, Shullman, & Gerlach, 1981). These regulations on employment selection procedures provided legal considerations prompting many organizations to review not only their employment practices but also their performance appraisal efforts. In 1978 the *Uniform Guidelines on Employee Selection Procedures* replaced the requirements of four major federal enforcement agencies (EEOC, Department of Justice, Department of Labor, and Civil Service Commission— later renamed the Office of Personnel Management) and provided one consistent set of federal regulations (EEOC, 1978).

In 1980 the *Standards for Nursing Services* of the Joint Commission on Accreditation of Hospitals mandated performance evaluation as part of Standard II (JCAH, 1983): "The nursing department/service shall be organized to meet the nursing care needs of patients and to maintain established standards of nursing practice" (p. 116). The JCAH interpretation of this standard includes, among other items, the following special attention to performance appraisal:

A written evaluation of the performance of registered nurses and ancillary nursing personnel shall be made at the end of the probationary period and at a defined interval thereafter. An annual evaluation is recommended. The evaluations must be criteria-based and shall relate to the standards of performance specified in the individual's job description. Job descriptions for each position classification shall also delineate the functions, responsibilities, and specific qualifications of each classification, and shall be made available to nursing personnel at the time they are hired and when requested. Job descriptions shall be reviewed periodically and revised as needed to reflect current job requirements. (p. 117)

It was during this same decade that the authors' work with hospital clients led them to develop the Results-Oriented Performance Evaluation Program (ROPEP), described in these publications (Ganong & Ganong, 1974, 1976, 1980a, 1981).

Problems with performance appraisal in the past have been many. Some of them that the authors identified had to do with the awkward situation in which department heads and nurse managers might find themselves. They know they are required or expected to evaluate the employees they supervise. But they often are frustrated, uncomfortable, even hostile to the whole routine:

- They find the existing evaluation procedure is inadequate for its purpose.
- They regard the techniques for evaluation as unsatisfactory for measuring results.
- They (the managers) are not sufficiently familiar with the performance of the person being evaluated.
- They lack training in the necessary interviewing and counseling skills.
- They have insufficient time to do evaluations.
- Their guilt feelings about all this tend to make them angry with the people they must evaluate.

What managers want from a performance appraisal system and what they get from it frequently are two different things. Managers expect and hope that appraisals will (1) effectively measure employee competence and (2) enrich the employee's experience in the job. However, research indicates that the majority of appraisal systems are neither effective nor valid for either purpose (Olmos, 1979).

Over a period of years the Center for Creative Leadership in Greensboro, N.C., has carried out an extensive survey of the literature on performance appraisal and the practices of a wide variety of organizations, culminating in the publication *Performance Appraisal on the Line* (DeVries et al., 1981).

They report several ways to define performance appraisal. One is to cite what the experts in the literature suggest should be happening under the guise of performance appraisal. Another is to describe the basic cognitive and interpersonal processes underlying this complex phenomenon. The definition they decided upon flows from how organizations currently view performance appraisal: "Performance appraisal is . . . the process by which an organization measures and evaluates an individual employee's behavior and accomplishments for a finite time period" (p. 2).

DeVries et al. find that performance appraisal has expanded considerably over the past quarter century to include such uses as: administrative decisions (salary, promotion, retention/discharge), counseling, training and development, human resources planning, and validation of selection techniques. It is clear that organizations' policies and practices for performance appraisal vary widely. Health care organizations probably are no better or worse in this regard than industry generally. Nursing departments in particular have shown commendable leadership in their efforts to refine and improve performance appraisal techniques.

PERFORMANCE APPRAISAL AS A MANAGEMENT TECHNIQUE

Performance evaluation is only one management technique (albeit a most important one) among many used by managers to carry out their functions of planning, doing, and controlling. Management techniques are used within a framework for management of a particular organization or department. A framework, by definition, is a basic system or design. (Figure 1-1 is an example.)

Nonnursing readers can readily adapt this framework to their own organizational situations. Implicit in the framework, and vital to it, are statements of the organization's mission, philosophy, goals, objectives, policies, procedures, and related documents and operational evidence that reflect the nature of its leadership. As experienced managers will acknowledge, the character of administrative leadership exhibited by the chief executive officer (CEO) is a greater determinant in creating a top performance climate than the mechanistic use of particular management techniques by department heads and supervisors.

Figure 1-1 A Framework for Nursing Management

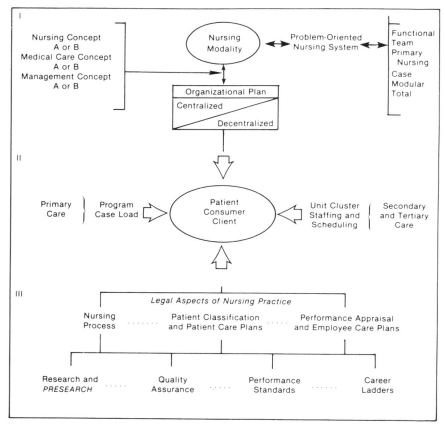

Source: Reprinted from *HELP with Managerial Leadership in Nursing: 101 Tremendous Trifles* (3rd ed.) by Joan M. Ganong and Warren L. Ganong with permission of W.L. Ganong Co., © 1980b, p. 41.

The success of performance appraisal, therefore, depends greatly upon its interrelationship with the other components of the framework for nursing management. This becomes even more evident as 15 criteria for an effective performance appraisal process are examined next in detail.

CRITERIA FOR AN EFFECTIVE PERFORMANCE APPRAISAL PROCESS

1. The purpose is clearly identified.

Too often this purpose is not stated and/or communicated. For example, Tosti (1980) lists 20 possible purposes of performance appraisal divided into either summative or formative categories (Table 1-1). Tosti's research indicates that each of these two forms of feedback obeys quite different rules. The differences may account for many of the problems in both formal and informal assessment systems.

Tosti defines formative feedback as the process by which information derived from either the process or the outcome is used to correct, guide, or modify the form of the behavior. Summative feedback is the process by which information derived from either the process or outcome is used to maintain or modify the likelihood or frequency of the behavior.

2. The process builds upon findings of the behavioral sciences—what is known about people and organizations.

The findings are extensive. Particularly pertinent are those in the fields of behavioristic, cognitive, and humanistic psychology. Readers of the management and behavioral science literature may recognize the contributions of such writers as Argyris, Bakke, Barnard, Bennis, Brown, Drucker, Erikson, Festinger, Freud, Friedman, Haire, Herzberg, Levitt, Lewin, Likert, Mager, Maslow, McClelland, McGregor, Myers, Roethlisberger, Rogers, Schein, Skinner, Yalom.

Table 1-1 Purposes of Performance Appraisal

Summative Purposes	*Formative Purposes*
Motivation	Career counseling
Pay increases	Work improvement
Termination	Eligibility for "growth" assignments
Promotions	Training
Reassignments	Individual development
Layoffs	Cross-training
Providing knowledge of output	Quality control
Select for a job	Scheduling
Problem prevention	Problem correction
Clarify accountability	Clarify job duties

Source: Reprinted from "The Sequential Feedback Model for Performance Assessment" by Donald Tosti: in *Job Performance Standards and Measures*, J.W. Springer (Ed.), with permission of the American Society for Training and Development, © 1980, p. 108.

3. It helps satisfy basic human needs.

The hierarchy of needs are physiological (survival), safety and security, love and belongingness, esteem, and self-actualization (Maslow, 1970). Typical performance appraisal plans in the past seem to have been designed deliberately to violate—or at the very least disregard—what is known about human needs and motivation.

For example, the appraisal forms often focus on weaknesses and short-comings and what must be done to improve them rather than on strengths and how to capitalize on them. Justification for such forms and practices usually has to do with equal employment opportunity regulations, building up a case for employees who should be transferred or discharged, and a host of other legal or otherwise similarly justifiable protective measures. The outcome, however, is continuing dissatisfaction with the end results. There has to be a better way, and there is.

4. The process can be adapted to individual differences.

Differences include all the factors of culture, economics, family, health, personal goals and objectives, talents, knowledge, skills, personality, religion, attitudes, and values. Recognizing such individual differences and the evidence of discriminatory practices in the past, legal restraints and personnel policies have been designed with the intent of treating all persons fairly by treating them equally.

In the authors' view, this is misguided. Treating people *equally* is no guarantee of treating them all *fairly* because, on the face of it, people are so different. The well-designed and well-implemented performance appraisal program takes into account individual differences. One of the ways to do so is to use employee care plans and to integrate the performance appraisal program with such plans.

5. The process focuses on strengths of individuals, not their weaknesses.

Over the years Peter Drucker has emphasized the fact that one can build only upon the strengths of individuals.

> The *development of a manager* focuses on the person. Its aim is to enable a man to develop his abilities and strengths to the fullest extent and to find individual achievement. The aim is excellence. . . . The starting point for any manager-development effort is a performance appraisal focused on what a man does well, what he can do well, and what limitations to his performance

capacity he needs to overcome to get the most out of his strengths. Such an appraisal, however, should always be a joint effort. It requires work on the part of the man himself; it has to be self-appraisal. But it also requires active leadership by a man's manager. . . . The question should always be asked, 'What are the right job experiences for this man so that his strengths can develop the fastest and the furthest?' (Drucker, 1974, pp. 426–427).

A manager the authors know made the same point in discussing one of his people who was holding a particularly sensitive position: "As long as his assets outweigh his liabilities I will continue him in his position. He is a known quantity, whereas another person whom I might hire or transfer will be a relatively unknown quantity in that position."

One unit director in a children's hospital writes:

> Over the years my approach to inclusion of negative comments in evaluations has changed based on the following premise. . . . Overall, all individuals have contributed to a unit as a whole. Their strengths may be diverse, with some contributing in more noticeable ways; however, collectively, a balance of strength is achieved and unit goals are met. Generally, limitations are minute in comparison to strengths and daily individual contributions. (Carlin, 1982)

Another writer (Wright, 1982) says:

> [M]anagers who succeed best are those who recognize that the average human has a fundamental capacity to do what needs to be done and to learn from experience. It is on this capacity that every skill is built. Competence is normal. Not only do humans have the ability to do well, they want to do well. Indeed, they *need* to do well, for it is by demonstrating competence that they build both self-respect and the respect of others.

The performance appraisal system needs to recognize the principles involved here and in so doing utilize the process for morale-building rather than morale-destroying purposes.

6. The system relates individual performance results with work unit goals and objectives.

This criterion would seem to be self-evident. Yet unless the performance appraisal process is deliberately designed to incorporate this item, one of the most significant purposes of the entire process can go unrealized.

7. The process measures performance results, not personal characteristics.

Personal traits and characteristics are important. They may well be identified as part of the specifications when recruiting and hiring people for particular jobs. But there is little to be gained, with rare exceptions, by evaluating trait-related factors in the appraisal process.

8. It utilizes mutually developed (understood and agreed-upon) standards of performance.

This is a key element in the initial development of an appraisal program. One of the main benefits of following this criterion is that both the superior and subordinate who are involved in the development of the standards of performance come away from the experience with a better understanding of the job activity itself and of what is expected in terms of results.

In addition, because of participation in developing the standards of performance, the participants will be much more committed to their use and to supporting the outcomes. Similar benefits are achieved with each new employee through an orientation with much emphasis on all aspects of the pertinent job performance description, including the performance standards.

9. It provides opportunity for accurate self-evaluation of performance.

When employees are invited to evaluate their own performance before an appraisal session with the boss, they may well be more critical of their performance than the superior. For example, studies and experience show that, in the supervisors' estimation, as many as 25 percent of employees underrate themselves, about 10 percent overrate themselves, and about 60 percent rate themselves approximately the same as do their superiors.

Accurate self-evaluation is most likely to occur with jointly developed standards of performance as described here. This approach shows respect for employees' knowledge and opinions about their jobs. It promotes the concept that true accountability and responsibility are within each individual (Albanese, 1975).

10. The process is carried out independently of wage and salary considerations.

When performance appraisal is used as the basis for annual wage adjustments, the temptation is great for the manager to slant the evaluation with budgetary considerations in mind. In fact, in one hospital the managers were instructed not to evaluate their people above the midpoint level because of budget restraints for that year.

From a practical standpoint, a wide variety of factors influence wages and salaries: length of service, supply and demand, competition, ability to pay (employer's financial condition), wage and price controls, labor unions, philosophy of the organization as interpreted by management, personal preferences, the fringe benefit package, and the entity's current goals and priorities.

In the final analysis, techniques such as job evaluation and employee evaluation are methods for assisting managers in establishing a fair day's pay for a fair day's work. They help to narrow the range of judgment within which a manager has to make decisions affecting each employee's pay. To that extent, these techniques and others like them can be useful.

Some organizations, however, have a policy of disassociating performance appraisal from the process of setting wages and salaries. This is in recognition of the influence of the aforementioned factors that dictate changes in wages from year to year. Such a policy permits performance appraisal to take place in an atmosphere free of the concerns related to pay adjustments. The major focus of attention then can be the performance of the employee in carrying out the job duties and responsibilities and how the individual and the superior evaluate the results.

The value of the performance appraisal process is diluted when it is viewed as a major determinant of wage adjustments. Performance appraisal should not be confused with merit rating but it can be used constructively for both summative and formative evaluation purposes and can influence employment status. This is accomplished best through a progressive wage and salary administration plan.

Such a plan is one that has an expanded number of steps on several career ladders and provides maximum opportunities for those who qualify to cross over from one track to another without penalty in terms of pay. The job classification for each level on each career track is the maximum rate that can be obtained through the job evaluation process. The specifications for being promoted to each level are clearly developed and shared so that employees know how they can qualify for promotion to the higher level.

The performance appraisal determines on a simple yes-or-no rating scale whether the person is satisfactory or unsatisfactory for each key element of the job performance description. When judged "satisfactory" on all (or 85 to 90 percent) of the major job performance responsibilities, the person deserves top-of-the-range pay in today's economic climate. Career ladders are presented in Chapter 6, with examples in the Appendixes.

This type of program puts a premium on all aspects of human resources management, including recruitment, hiring, orientation, staff development, retention, continuing education, on-the-job training, performance appraisal, and related considerations.

11. The system facilitates agreement on evaluation outcomes between superior and subordinate.

This criterion is fulfilled almost automatically when the program is carried out as designed. The features of mutually developed standards of performance and the self-evaluation by each person using these measures lead to greater understanding and agreement in the appraisal process.

12. The process is economical to use.

Economical as used here is a function not only of time invested in development and implementation but also the side effects of the use of a plan. A cheaply designed system of performance appraisal may well be a highly expensive investment if the plan does not well serve the intended purposes or if the side effects include lower morale and less-than-satisfactory on-the-job results.

A substantial start-up cost can be justified if there is evidence that the system will be well accepted, used for its intended purposes, and contribute to quality assurance and cost control.

13. The process adheres to organizational philosophy, and to pertinent governmental or contractual requirements from a legal standpoint.

The performance appraisal system needs to reinforce rather than dilute the organization's philosophy and mission. Pertinent governmental and contractual regulations must be adhered to both legally and ethically. These are to be considered not as constraints that limit the viability of a program but rather as guidelines within which it must operate.

14. The system uses a simple OK/NOT-OK (satisfactory/unsatisfactory) appraisal of results for each key performance responsibility.

Why use measures of "satisfactory" performance instead of some higher goal of excellence? Perhaps the reasons are already evident. They include:

- being realistic as to what level of performance should be expected as a "fair day's work for a fair day's pay"

- the demanding nature of the "satisfactory" standard, especially when the measure is "no errors" in the critical tasks of patient care
- the managers' and supervisors' having learned through experience the fallacies and hazards of more complicated appraisal methods
- the consistency of such evaluation with labor union philosophy and practice as well as with sound personnel administration policy
- the excellence in performance that often occurs in spite of, not because of, an appraisal program designed as a management control system to achieve it; excellence is achieved by people with pride in their work, who get satisfaction from it.

Such an OK/NOT-OK evaluation scale has the benefits of being easy to use, facilitating agreement, taking a minimum amount of time, and being viewed by all concerned as common sense in the context of the entire human resources management system. It is supported by other references, including Schwind (1980). Other versions of simple evaluation scales are included in other chapters and the appendixes.

15. **The process emphasizes the achievement of mutual understanding and agreement rather than the trained use of particular evaluation instruments and forms.**

Performance appraisal needs to be seen as a human rather than a technical process. The system used should focus on achieving the highest degree of mutual understanding possible between superior and subordinate in terms of what is expected by way of on-the-job performance and results and how to achieve and/or maintain a satisfactory level of performance and results.

These 15 criteria serve well the subject of this book—*Performance Appraisal for Productivity: the nurse manager's role*. The focus turns now to productivity.

PRODUCTIVITY AND THE NURSE MANAGER

Productivity is the noun form of the adjective "productive." Productive is defined as (1) producing or capable of producing; (2) producing abundantly; fertile, prolific; (3) yielding favorable or useful results; constructive; (4) in economics, of or involved in the creation of goods and services to produce wealth or value (American Heritage, 1973).

In everyday language productivity is a measure of what people get out for what they put in—input vs. output. The concept is simple to understand. However, it is not so simple when nurse managers are asked to contribute to achieving increasingly favorable productivity results in their areas of responsibility and accountability. These results often are expressed as a single productivity measure, with progress noted from day to day, week by week, and month to month.

In nursing, the ultimate bottom-line figure is the cost per patient day or cost per other measurable unit of service such as number of procedures performed, weighted according to degree of difficulty. Other hospital departments use similar measures, depending upon their types of service that, when combined, provide the hospital's own bottom line in terms of cost per patient day for each month. By itself this is a rough and sometimes misleading performance measure for the facility, particularly when used for interhospital comparisons.

Research in recent years has provided what has become a more acceptable basis for analyzing hospital costs and productivity and as a basis for prospective reimbursement. This is the development of the Diagnosis-Related Groups (DRGs)—that are the measure that rewards hospitals with favorable comparisons and penalizes those with less favorable figures (Grimaldi & Micheletti, 1982a). The role of nurse managers has become even more significant—and recognized as such—in affecting the 24-hour cost of operation of the hospital system. This is because nurse managers are the single most important group integrating the day in, day out, round-the-clock operation of the facility.

Performance appraisal provides a vital link between the largest single supervisory group in the hospital (the nurse managers) and the single largest group of its employees (the hourly paid, nonexempt employees on the nursing department payroll). Nurse managers thus have a profound effect on the productivity of the organization through their skills in carrying out the nursing management functions and techniques.

The management functions are those of planning, doing, and controlling (Ganong & Ganong, 1980a). The management techniques referred to include:

- developing job performance descriptions that describe measures of productivity (quality and quantity performance criteria) for each key job responsibility and/or duty
- performance appraisal based on those job performance descriptions
- merit rating when desirable as a basis for wage and salary adjustments
- career ladders on the management, education, research, and clinical tracks with defined levels based upon the job performance descriptions

- the related techniques of management by objectives, quality assurance, staffing and scheduling, and annual budgetary planning (Ganong & Ganong, 1980a).

Performance appraisal in the modern sense—not just as an annual or semiannual time-consuming event—embraces the day-to-day process of observation, coaching, and guidance that encourages and permits individuals to exhibit their natural tendencies toward competent performance (Wright, 1982). After all, true accountability is within oneself. When every employee recognizes and believes this fact, productivity is influenced for the better. Performance appraisal, providing for both summative and formative feedback, is a key nursing management tool and a technique for improving productivity.

The regular performance review and appraisal provides an opportunity for all employees to let the superior know how they think they are doing individually and for the manager to agree or disagree as appropriate. This apparently simple and potentially satisfying communication process becomes complicated and distasteful when it becomes overly structured and formalized.

Productivity Formulas

Two dictionary definitions of the word "formula" apply here. One is "a mathematical statement, especially an equation, of a rule, principle, answer, or other logical relation" (American Heritage, 1973). The second is "a conventionalized statement intended to express some fundamental truth" (Merriam-Webster, 1971). Thus a formula may be a mathematically precise equation or a less precise, but nonetheless useful, expression of relationships that can help with a manager's most important skill—conceptualizing, the mental process of developing a concept, plan, design, idea, or thought.

Productivity formulas typically express an input/output relationship. More specifically, the concept is that of input and throughput leading to measurable output/outcome. One version of such a formula is as follows:

$$M^1 + M^2 + M^3 = R^1$$

This shows how the resources of M^1—manpower (people), M^2—materials (supplies), and M^3—machines (equipment) when added together in a suitable combination produce a given level of productive results (R^1). R^1 may be the number of days of patient care, number of laboratory tests or Xrays per day, pounds of laundry per week, meals per month, or whatever units are appropriate.

Varying the measurable amount of any one of the Ms on the input side of the formula might be expected to have a corresponding influence on the quantity and quality of the results (R^1) on the output side. However, experienced managers know that it is not quite that simple. They know that the caliber of managerial leadership has a great deal to do with the utilization of available resources and strongly influences the output side of the formula. Thus this particular productivity formula becomes fully meaningful only when it includes the Big M^4 for Management:

$$M^4(M^1 + M^2 + M^3) = R^2$$

The *M*-for-Manager is shown not as just another addition to the formula but as a multiplying factor. The manager's influence on results (R^2) is pervasive. It permeates everything else, magnifying the outcomes, usually for the better, sometimes not. When the manager provides strong and effective managerial leadership, the productivity results are multiplied rather than simply being added to. Less effective managerial leadership correspondingly provides a significant negative influence on the quality and quantity of the results.

The fifth M in what becomes the 5-M formula is money. This can be included in the formula by adding a dollar sign over each of the other elements.

Money becomes the least common denominator for all of the other elements. It is the unit of measure used for the organization's financial statement. A dollars-and-cents figure provides the bottomline measure for the operating results of the input/output process.

Other output reports are essential, too. These are the outcomes in human terms—the quantity/quality/personal data that identify how well the agency is fulfilling its human-service goals. Are these more important than the financial measures? The answer is neither yes nor no because both are essential—the money and the service to people. One does not exist without the other. Adequate financing and a controlled budget are essential if services are to be provided at any level of quality and quantity.

Admittedly some managers are better than others at getting the maximum units of service (quality and quantity) out of each dollar of operating expense. One reason for this is their skill in both individual and group relations (Ganong & Ganong, 1980a, p. 295–302). And a vital aspect of using such skill is the technique of performance appraisal that they use.

Assessing Worker Contribution to Productivity

Exhibit 1-1 is another productivity formula that includes elements some-times overlooked (Sharplin & Mondy, 1982). This provides a framework for evaluating worker contribution to organizational productivity. The worker's own contribution is indeed a most important one but too often, it has been the only one considered.

As shown in the equation, however, another important element is the employee's contribution to the performance of coworkers. This is indi-cated as a plus-or-minus factor. It is a plus factor when the individual employee sets a good example through personal productivity and behavior or perhaps by finding other ways of contributing to the performance of fellow workers. It is a negative influence when the employee's behavior (extra socializing, poor teamwork) interferes with the others' performance.

Clearly, any behavior that makes a worker's contribution to the pro-ductivity of others less than it reasonably could be is the proper concern of the manager. It can be dealt with most effectively in day-to-day on-the-job guidance rather than being left to the formal appraisal session.

The amount of supervision required is the final element in this equation. It is shown as a negative factor since, when the amount of supervision required is least, the unit productivity results are the highest. Spending excessive time with an employee tends to distract the manager from other duties and opportunities for productivity improvement.

Whether a worker *is* a problem or *has* a problem, a supervisor's overriding concern should be with unit productivity. It is not enough to consider individual output. An employee's impact on

Exhibit 1-1 Assessing Worker Contribution to the Work Unit

Assessing Worker Contribution to the Work Unit

Worker's Contribution to Productivity	=	Quality & Quantity of Work Done	±	Contribution to the Performance of Other Employees	−	Amount of Supervision Required

Source: Reprinted from "Looking Beyond Individual Productivity" by A.D. Sharplin and R.W. Mondy in *Supervisory Management,* November 1982, *27* (11), p. 4, with permission of the authors, the publisher.

other workers is just as important. Finally, good supervisory talent is a rare and precious commodity in most organizations. The degree to which a worker uses that commodity also affects work unit productivity. These three elements should be considered in a relatively hard-nosed fashion in designing methods to improve productivity and correct patterns of employee misbehavior. (Sharplin & Mondy, 1982, p. 5)

A Productivity Index

A more sophisticated productivity index formula is provided by Hanson (1982):

Productivity index = Production % × Resource utilization %

Hanson describes how to calculate the production percentage by dividing utilized resources by required units of production (required resources). The resource utilization percentage is obtained by dividing utilized resources by purchased resources. Hanson uses hours of service as the measure of both resources and units of production:

- Required units of production (required resources) is the required hours of service based on studies, philosophy, and professional judgment.
- Purchased resources is the hours of personnel time acquired.
- Available resources equals purchased resources multiplied by resource effectiveness.
- Utilized resources is the lesser of available resources or required units of production.
- Provided units of production equals utilized resources.

Hanson (1982) points out that defining the key element of resource effectiveness depends on how human resources are defined. From the variety of possible definitions, he has selected four elements of human resources in the following formula:

Resource effectiveness = % knowledge and skill × % energy (physical, mental, emotional) × % motivation × % self-directedness

Hanson continues with examples of how the concepts and formulas can be applied toward maximizing the utilization of human resources to achieve the most production. He offers 11 exhibits in a case study that assumes that the required product be six hours of service per patient. These hours are broken down into four hours of professional (Type A) and two hours of nonprofessional (Type B) services.

He shows how the nurse administrator can cope in various ways when faced with a cost cutback situation. His detailed analyses of various options provide an excellent cost/benefit comparison of the possibilities. Reading of the entire article is recommended. Hanson concludes:

> The fiscal resources available to nursing administrators for the acquisition of human resources may be largely outside our direct control and indeed in the years to come may force us to face cutback realities. How we choose to manage these limited fiscal resources, however, is within our control and will depend on our ability to analyze, interpret, and respond to varied conditions and potentials for production, resource utilization, and productivity. Unless we make the proper decisions, the old adage "penny wise and pound foolish" could easily become the description of nursing reality. (p. 23)

DRGs and RIMs

All of the foregoing analysis takes on additional relevance when considered in the light of the federal government's prospective payment system (PPS) for Medicare that mandates change from a per diem basis to a cost-per-discharge system (TEFRA, 1982). With such a system, the hospital is not reimbursed for the number of days a patient stays in the facility but rather a specific predetermined amount of money is allocated to each patient according to the medical diagnosis.

> The cornerstone of the government's new prospective payment plan is the Diagnostic Related Groups (DRG) concept originally developed at Yale University as a management and utilization review tool. To put it simply, the patient population is divided into Major Diagnostic Categories (MDCs) which are further subdivided into 356 Diagnostic Related Groupings (DRGs) subdivided according to age and the presence or absence of complications. A dollar figure, based upon retrospective costs data for a hospital and region, is derived by averaging the cost of the care given to patients who have had this diagnosis, adjusted, presumably, to account for inflation plus 1%. A hospital's income for Medicare (and undoubtedly eventually Medicaid) will be determined by dividing the allowable Medicare costs assigned to each

DRG by the number of patients discharged who have been assigned
to that DRG. What this means in plain language is that hospitals
must cut their costs by millions more than originally projected.
(Curtin, 1982, p. 7)

The original basis for apportioning nursing costs among the DRGs, and
for calculating the amount paid for nursing care, were patient days. Taking
note of dissatisfaction among nurses with the per diem method, the New
Jersey Department of Health initiated studies to develop another way for
allocating nursing costs. Relative intensity measures (RIMs) are one of
these. "Total nursing costs—essentially the salaries and fringe benefits
paid to registered nurses, licensed practical nurses, and nurse aides—
comprise roughly 30 percent of the typical hospital's budget for direct
patient care. Therefore, proper allocation of nursing costs is essential if
the hospital costs are to be measured accurately" (Grimaldi & Micheletti,
1982b, p. 12).

The impact of all of this on the affected hospitals will be great. (Those
not subject to the limits include most rural hospitals of fewer than 50 beds;
long-term care hospitals, i.e., those whose average length of stay is greater
than 30 days; and children's hospitals.) Nursing departments will be especially affected as the pressure increases to reduce costs. Curtin (1982)
believes that the impact on nursing can produce one of two results:

(1) Hospitals may return to a system which allows only one or
two registered nurses for 30–50 patients (outside the intensive
care units). Nurses themselves would perform few clinical functions; rather they would coordinate and supervise the activities
of technicians. (2) Hospitals may cut down on or eliminate many
support services and nurses will give *total* care to patients—no
more pharmacy techs to give medication; no more respiratory
techs to give Bennet treatments; no more IV techs to put in and
take out IVs, and so forth. (p. 8)

THE OUTLOOK

Fortunately, over the past decade or so nursing management has taken
great strides. Head nurses, supervisors, and others in nursing administration have demonstrated that, given the tools to work with and the training
in how to use them, they are among the very best managers in the health
care industry.

The Joint Commission on Accreditation of Hospitals (JCAH) (1983) has
contributed to this end with its updated standards for nursing service.

Many well-designed patient classification systems already are in place. They will continue to be refined, many being adapted for computer systems as part of a hospital management information system. Continued refinements and advances in hospital computer systems will be necessary to keep track of the tremendous volume of statistics and to help facilities avoid the financial penalties for exceeding the predetermined reimbursement amounts for each of the DRGs.

In all of this the role of the nurse managers will be paramount, and never more so than in their skillful utilization of the performance appraisal process as a continuing technique for optimal productivity.

For Discussion Purposes

As members of a performance appraisal task force for the nursing department, you have been asked to evaluate all aspects of your present performance appraisal program. You can find no clear statement of purpose for the appraisal program, and decide that this is the first task to accomplish.

1. Describe how you would begin to identify the purposes for your performance appraisal program. Consider whom to include in this process, both in and outside the nursing department.
2. Identify what other aspects of nursing management and hospital administration must be considered.
3. Decide what to do to achieve a consensus, especially if there appears to be a division of opinion as to the scope of purposes to be served by performance appraisal.

NOTES

Albanese, R. *Management: Toward accountability for performance.* Homewood, Ill.: Richard D. Irwin, Inc., 1975.

The American heritage dictionary of the English language. New York: Dell Publishing Co., Inc., 1973.

American Hospital Association. *Employee performance appraisal programs: Guidelines for the development and implementation.* Chicago: Author, 1971.

Carlin, B.J. Work evaluations are effective if . . . *Nursing Management,* September 1982, *13*(9), 10.

Curtin, L. The new federal regs: Survival and revival. *Nursing Management,* December 1982, *13*(12), 7–8.

DeVries, D.L.; Morrison, A.M.; Shullman, S.L.; & Gerlach, M.L. *Performance appraisal on the line.* New York: John Wiley & Sons, Inc., 1981.

Drucker, P.F. *Management: tasks, responsibilities, practices.* New York: Harper & Row, Publishers, Inc., 1974.

Drucker, P.F. *Managing in turbulent times.* New York: Harper & Row, Publishers, Inc., 1980.

Equal Employment Opportunity Commission. Uniform guidelines on employee selection procedures. *Federal Register,* August 25, 1978, *43*(166), 38290–38309.

Ganong, J.M., & Ganong, W.L. *HELP* with a results-oriented performance evaluation program.* Chapel Hill, N.C.: W.L. Ganong Co., 1974.

Ganong, J.M., & Ganong, W.L. *Nursing management.* Rockville, Md.: Aspen Systems Corporation, 1976.

Ganong, J.M., & Ganong, W.L. *Nursing management* (2nd ed.). Rockville, Md.: Aspen Systems Corporation, 1980. (a)

Ganong, J.M., & Ganong, W.L. *HELP with Managerial Leadership in Nursing: 101 Tremendous Trifles* (3rd ed.). Chapel Hill, N.C.: W.L. Ganong Co., 1980. (b)

Ganong, J.M. & Ganong, W.L. *HELP with performance appraisal.* Chapel Hill, N.C.: W.L. Ganong Co., 1981.

Grimaldi, P.L., & Micheletti, J.A. *DRGs: A practitioner's guide.* Chicago: Pluribus Press, 1982. (a)

Grimaldi, P.L., & Micheletti, J.A. RIMs and the cost of nursing care. *Nursing Management,* December 1982, *13*(12), 12. (b)

Hanson, R.L. Managing human resources. *The Journal of Nursing Administration,* December 1982, *12*(12), 17–23.

Joint Commission on Accreditation of Hospitals. *Accreditation manual for hospitals.* Chicago: Author, 1983.

Lewin, K. *Field theory and social science.* New York: Harper & Brothers, 1951.

Likert, R. *The human organization: Its management and value.* New York: McGraw-Hill Book Company, 1967.

Mager, R. *Developing attitude toward learning.* Belmont, Calif.: Fearon, Lear Sigler, 1968.

Marriner, A. (Ed.). *Current perspectives in nursing management.* St. Louis: The C.V. Mosby Company, 1979.

Maslow, A. *Motivation and personality* (2nd ed.). New York: Harper & Row, Publishers, Inc., 1970.

McGregor, D. *The human side of enterprise.* New York: McGraw-Hill Book Company, 1960.

Myers, M.S. *Every employee a manager.* New York: McGraw-Hill Book Company, 1970.

Olmos, S. Employees help to define their jobs. *Hospitals,* June 16, 1979, *53*(12), 79–81.

Ornstein, R. *The psychology of consciousness.* San Francisco: W.H. Freeman & Co., 1972.

Ouchi, W. *Theory Z.* Reading Mass.: Addison-Wesley Publishing Company, 1981.

Rogers, C. *Freedom to learn.* Columbus, Ohio: The Charles E. Merrill Publishing Co., Inc., 1969.

Rogers, C., & Stevens, B. *Person to person: The problem of being human.* New York: Pocket Books, Inc., 1971.

Rokeach, M. *The nature of human values.* New York: The Free Press, 1973.

---

* The HELP acronym is for Health Education and Learning Program. There have been 20 titles in the HELP series of Nursing Management Guides.

Schwind, H.F. Behavior sampling for effective performance feedback. In J. Springer (Ed.), *Job performance standards and measures*. Madison, Wis.: American Society for Training and Development, 1980.

Sharplin, A.D., & Mondy, R.W. Looking beyond individual productivity. *Supervisory Management,* November 1982, *27*(11), 3–9.

Stevens, B. *The Nurse as executive.* Rockville, Md.: Aspen Systems Corporation, 1975.

Tax Equity and Fiscal Responsibility Act of 1982 (TEFRA) (P.L. 97-248). Washington, D.C.: U.S. Government Printing Office.

Tosti, D. The sequential feedback model for performance assessment. In J. Springer (Ed.), *Job performance standards and measures* (Paper No. 4, ASTD Research Series). Madison, Wis.: American Society for Training and Development, 1980.

Webster's new collegiate dictionary (8th ed.). Springfield, Mass.: Merriam-Webster, 1981.

Wright, J. Is competence normal? *Data Forum,* Fall 1982, *1*(1).

Reading List

Argyris, C. *Personality and organization.* New York: Harper & Row, 1957.

Bakke, E.W. *Teamwork in industry.* (Labor & Management Center, Reprint No. 10), New Haven: Yale University, 1948.

Barnard, C. *The functions of the executive.* Cambridge, Mass.: Harvard University Press, 1938.

Bennis, W. *Changing organizations.* New York: McGraw-Hill Book Company, 1966.

Bennis, W.; Berlew, D.; Schein, E.; & Steele, F. *Interpersonal dynamics* (3rd ed.). Homewood, Ill.: The Dorsey Press, 1973.

Brown, G. *Human teaching for human learning.* New York: The Viking Press, 1971.

Drucker, P. *Management: Tasks, responsibilities, practices.* New York: Harper & Row, Publishers, Inc., 1973.

Erikson, E. *Identity and the life cycle.* New York: International Universities Press, 1959.

Friedman, W. *How to do groups.* New York: Jason Aronson, Inc., 1979.

Herzberg, F.; Mausner, B.; & Snyderman, B. *The motivation to work.* New York: John Wiley, & Sons, Inc., 1959.

McClelland, D.G., Atkinson, J.W., Clark, R.A., & Lowell, E.L. *The achievement motive.* New York: Appleton-Century-Crofts, Inc., 1953.

Yalom, I. *The theory and practice of group psychotherapy* (2nd ed.). New York: Basic Books, Inc., 1975.

Chapter 2

Performance Appraisal Research

BACKGROUND, ASSUMPTIONS AND REALITIES

The past several decades have seen a proliferation of books and articles about performance appraisal. Many of these have stemmed from soundly based research, studies, surveys, and the experiences of individuals and specific organizations. A review of these materials can be a sobering experience. This chapter provides a selective summary of some of their pertinent findings.

An Easier Look at Performance Appraisal (Beaulieu, 1980) helps bring the subject into focus. Beaulieu begins with a brief comment about the oft-quoted article *An Uneasy Look at Performance Appraisal* (McGregor, 1957), in which McGregor recommended that employees be appraised on the basis of short-term performance goals, rather than traits, that are set jointly by the employee and the manager. Then Beaulieu writes:

> In spite of the bramble bushes that now cover empirical trails of systems installed, blandly ignored, and ultimately abandoned, the legend of the immense benefits to be derived from employee evaluation still persists in the minds and hearts of executives. Like aged prospectors who wearily search the mountains pursuing dreams of buried treasures, personnel folk pour over forms, seek new substitutes for old cliches, attend workshops, and sometimes come up with a "system" that, with a lot of luck and the appropriate signatures, gets "sold" to people in the organization.

Beaulieu cites the most massive entry into the field of mandated performance appraisals as that of the federal government with its *Civil Service Reform Act of 1978* (P.L. 95-454). That provides for a system of performance standards with employee evaluation to determine their eligibility for merit pay increases and promotions. This well-motivated but expensive venture has produced mixed results. The authors can sympathize with Beaulieu's statements because of their involvement with one segment of the federal government in this effort.

As Beaulieu points out, using a performance appraisal system successfully as one of the means toward the end of increased organizational productivity need not be excessively expensive nor cumbersome. But before that can happen, the people who are interested in making that occur must shed some *erroneous* assumptions and confront several realities. Five of these erroneous assumptions and the concomitant reality about each can be summarized (based on Beaulieu) as follows:

> *Assumption No. 1:* Managers have a clear sense of organizational direction and can readily fit expectations of employee performance into that framework.

Reality: Most managers have, at best, a blurred perception of where they want their organizations to go. They tend, and perhaps prefer, to operate in a crisis/reactive state rather than follow predefined paths of progress (Mintzberg, 1973).

What is needed of course is to oblige managers to prepare a written business plan that lists priorities, goals, and strategies. Preparing such a plan should be part of the manager's evaluation. Once the plan is prepared and endorsed by higher management it brings general expectations of employees much more sharply into focus.

> *Assumption No. 2:* In preparing performance standards, managers will begin with position descriptions or other devices that objectively and impersonally describe job responsibilities.

Reality: Most job descriptions, if they exist at all and are not hopelessly out of date, list job activities rather than accomplishments. Some of the drawbacks of the typical job description include: failing to overlap very much with what an employee actually does; too often written by a manager considering only the characteristics of individual employee; providing inconsistent standards, lack of challenge; leaving manager vulnerable to charges of various kinds of discrimination.

These limitations make it practically impossible to link evaluations with merit pay and promotional opportunity. The solution is for managers to be sure the job description is as up to date as possible, then to relate it to the business plan and identify several accomplishments that an ideal employee would generate.

Assumption No. 3: Any experienced manager can readily identify employee competence; hence, written performance standards ought not to be difficult.

Reality: Most managers are not well equipped to *define* competence, much less recognize it (Gilbert, 1978). Gilbert relates competence to accomplishments, and describes them as the worthy results that are visible after an employee goes home. Accomplishments should always form the basis of job standards.

Assumption No. 4: Performance standards, to be valid, must be completely measurable by quantifiable yardsticks.

Reality: The majority of critical performance elements simply cannot be viewed in pounds, dollars, liters, and other countable things. To limit performance standards to issues that readily accommodate a pure scorecard is to bypass much of what should be expected of an employee. Furthermore, "countability" frequently requires an impossible monitoring system. The illusive pursuit of ways to measure the unmeasurable is avoided when it is recognized that the locus is verification, not quantification. Means of verifying accomplishments are far easier to arrive at than are rigidly quantifiable measurements. The performance standard that eludes verification has not yet presented itself.

Assumption No. 5: Clearly written personnel bulletins, "how-to" pamphlets, exhortations from on high, and a one or two-day training session (which mostly presents all of the above), are all that is necessary to implant the system.

Reality: The whole issue is terribly complex, involves new and complicated mind sets, and requires managers to exercise mental muscles they are largely inexperienced in using. Fully adequate and extensive training and counseling support are necessary to bring about the self-confidence managers must have if there is any genuine expectation that beneficial performance appraisal programs ever will fly.

Beaulieu's strong conviction is that where performance evaluation is concerned, the past is not necessarily prologue. Perhaps managers have learned from their own mistakes. Perhaps the whole body of knowledge about the relationships of people to their jobs acquired in recent years, and a willingness to shift mental gears will guide managers to new thinking about an old idea. There really is buried treasure in those mountains, and the search is not futile. Merely difficult.

Beaulieu's common sense commentary is in keeping with our own experience and philosophy. For example, Beaulieu mentions an annual business plan requirement under discussion of Assumption No. 1. We described and recommended such a plan in our article *ABP for Nursing Administration* (Ganong & Ganong, 1973). It provided a model for our book *HELP with Annual Budgetary Planning* (Ganong & Ganong, 1976). As the ABP article said:

> An annual business plan for nursing service provides a coordinated, businesslike way for nursing service administration to plan, operate, and control the activities of its department. While most nursing service departments and their institutions have some elements of an ABP, too few nursing service administrators use all the elements as described as a basis for planning and decision making. And too few nursing service departments participate adequately in the preparation of an ABP when the institution itself uses such a plan. (p. 61)

That message was much less recognized a decade or so ago than it is today. The urgency now, however, is even greater in terms of recognizing the complexities of a performance evaluation program and structuring it sensibly so that it can be used effectively by nurse managers in their efforts toward achieving full productivity of their departmental units.

The foregoing provides an appropriate backdrop for considering some of the survey and research findings in the field.

'DECADE OF THE NURSE' SURVEY

In the fall of 1981 the authors surveyed readers of their *G-GRAM: Newsletter for Nurse Managers and Educators* (Vol. 8, No. 5), asking them to compare the situation in their own hospital (or agency) and region to what it had been two years earlier. Exhibit 2-1 summarizes responses from readers in 45 states.

Readers replied to the statement "Here's how I see nurses, and nursing, today as compared with two years ago in 1979," rating each of the ten factors listed. A clear majority, more than 50 percent, said that nurses were *better off* in respect to these five factors:

Exhibit 2-1 Survey of Changes in Nursing, 1979–1981

In Respect to:	A	B	C
1. Use of the Nursing Process	60	33	7
2. Clinical expertise of nsg. staff	65	27	8
3. Managerial expertise	58	29	13
4. Status in eyes of patients/public	30	57	13
5. Respect for nurses by physicians	32	54	14
6. Support of hosp./agency admin.	51	38	11
7. Job Satisfaction	29	47	24
8. Wages	63	21	16
9. Availability of BSN for working RN	35	49	16
10. Preparation of students to nurse:			
a) Diploma grads	18	55	27
b) Assoc. Degree grads	15	64	21
c) BSN graduates	24	60	16

Percent of Responses in Each Category

Coding: A=Better Off; B=About the same; C=Falling behind

Source: Reprinted from *The G-GRAM: Newsletter for Nurse Managers and Educators.* Special Report, November 1981, with permission of Warren L. Ganong and Joan M. Ganong, editors and publishers, © 1981.

1. use of the nursing process (60 percent)
2. clinical expertise of nursing staff (65 percent)
3. managerial expertise (58 percent)
6. support of hospital/agency administration (51 percent)
8. wages (63 percent)

The five other factors were all rated *about the same* by 47 percent to 64 percent of the respondents, as follows:

4. status in eyes of patients/public (57 percent)
5. respect for nurses by physicians (54 percent)
7. job satisfaction (47 percent)
9. availability of B.S.N. for working R.N. (49 percent)
10. preparation of students to nurse (55 percent to 64 percent)

The *falling behind* category ranged from 7 percent (for #1, Use of the nursing process) to 27 percent (for #10, Preparation of diploma graduates to nurse)—clearly a poor third place in the outcomes.

The position titles of director of nursing and assistant director of nursing predominated among the respondents. Next in order were other nurse manager titles, staff development directors, and other nurse educators. Some inserted additional factors in the Other listing (#11 on the survey form). Some of these, and the scores assigned, are:

- labor union activity (A)
- political action conscious (C)
- quality assurance (A)
- sense of professional vs. economic security (A)
- staff level involvement in planning and decision making (A)
- professional responsiveness and responsibility (C)
- awareness of nursing issues (A)
- turnover of personnel (C).

Many additional comments are available in the summary report (Ganong & Ganong, 1981). The diversity of opinions expressed was substantial, often because of a local situation.

In summary, it is clear that while individual opinions varied widely, the balance is on the side of, "We are *better off* (on the five primary factors) and at least *about the same* (on the five secondary factors) compared with two years ago." The authors concluded that nurses, especially nurse managers (in both practice and education settings) could continue the positive thrusts that justified their calling the 1980s "The Decade of the Nurse." In addition, the findings are informative in terms of some of the factors evaluated (managerial expertise, support of hospital administration, job satisfaction, and wages) having relevance to performance appraisal and productivity.

PERFORMANCE APPRAISAL SURVEY REPORT

In early 1982 the authors again surveyed newsletter readers, this time on their performance appraisal practices. Exhibit 2-2 summarizes the responses from a sampling of large and small hospitals in 34 states.

The high percentage of *Yes* responses (74 percent to 83 percent) to statements 1 through 3 reflects the efforts of nursing departments generally to improve performance appraisal practices and to use competency-based performance standards. Of the respondents, 55 percent use a results-oriented appraisal procedure, 44 percent provide for self-appraisal of performance, and 82 percent say that a usual outcome of the evaluation is a plan for further self-development and/or behavior change. Some 64 percent indicate less than full satisfaction with present appraisal procedures.

These findings reflect the tremendous time and effort devoted by nursing departments to updating performance appraisal procedures, stimulated largely by the interpretation of Standard II of the Joint Commission on Accreditation of Hospitals 1980 *Standards for Nursing Services* (see the

Exhibit 2-2 Performance Appraisal Survey Report

Survey questionnaires were mailed with our Jan/Feb '82 *G-GRAM* issue. So far, 66 responses have been received from a sampling of large and small hospitals in 34 states. Here is a quick summary showing the percent of YES and NO answers for each statement.

YES	NO	
83%	17%	1. We have revised our performance appraisal forms within past 3 years.
77	23	2. Our job descriptions are the basis for performance appraisal.
74	26	3. Job descriptions include standards of performance.
38	62	4. Our job description is used as the performance appraisal form.
33	67	5. We use a separate merit rating form.
68	32	6. We have a merit wage adjustment based upon merit rating.
55	45	7. We use a results-oriented performance appraisal procedure.
39	61	8. We use the same appraisal form for nurse managers as for staff RNs and other nursing department employees.
45	55	9. Other hospital departments use the same appraisal form as nursing.
15	85	10. Job descriptions & perform. appraisal are part of a career ladder program.
82	18	11. A usual outcome of performance appraisal is plan for self-development.
44	56	12. Our plan involves self-appraisal of one's own performance.
36	64	13. I am satisfied with our present performance appraisal procedure.
36	64	14. I am enclosing examples of job (performance) descriptions.

Source: Reprinted from *The G-GRAM: Newsletter for Nurse Managers and Educators,* 1982, 9(2), with permission of Warren L. Ganong and Joan M. Ganong, editors and publishers, © 1982.

beginning of Chapter 1, supra). The examples in the 13 appendixes show that the results of these efforts range from very simple and easy-to-use systems to others that are much more complex, ambitious, and time consuming.

The results of performance appraisal efforts in this sampling of the nation's hospitals deserve comparison with Beaulieu's "erroneous assumptions" and "realities" given at the beginning of this chapter. On balance, however, the strong responses of nursing departments to the JCAH Standard, as well as other efforts not directly stimulated by the JCAH, have been creative, professional, and reflect credit upon the nurses and other personnel involved. Once again the authors find justification for their long-held opinion that nurses comprise a higher percentage of the best managers in the health care field than any other professional group.

We expect this opinion to be further validated as nurses continue to contribute to the refinement of present performance appraisal programs and their use toward the goals of optimal productivity and quality of personnel performance.

EVALUATING NURSE ADMINISTRATORS

This section reports the findings of a doctoral research study of relationships among self-actualizing, tolerance of ambiguity, job stress, and performance track record as perceived by nurse administrators (Ganong, 1981). The operational definitions of key terms are:

Self-actualizing:
> The process used by well people to become more effective and self-fulfilled through identified values and behaviors.

Tolerance of Ambiguity:
> The tendency to perceive ambiguous situations as bearable.

Perceived Job Stress:
> Awareness of unpleasant psychological states evoked by threatening environmental events or stimuli in a general hospital work setting.

Nurse Administrator:
> The registered nurse who has responsibility for planning, directing, and controlling the hospital's department of nursing, including accountability for the quality of nursing care patients receive.

Perceived Performance Track Record:
> The cumulative work results of accomplishments and defeats, including consideration of resources, limitations, and values during the past year as perceived by the Nurse Administrator. (Ganong, 1981, p. 45)

The subjects were 84 nurse administrators in general hospitals of 100 to 600 beds selected by random sampling in 50 states.

The four instruments used for data collection, in addition to a demographic data sheet, included two personality measures: *The Personal Orientation Inventory* (POI) developed by Everett L. Shostrom (1964, 1968); and the *AT-20 for Tolerance of Ambiguity* (MacDonald, 1970).

The first of two performance measures used included job stress indexes developed by House, Wells, Landerman, McMichael, and Kaplan (1979). The five types of job stress assessed were responsibility pressure, quality concern, role conflict, job vs. nonjob conflict, and workload. The second performance measure is the *Perceived Performance Track Record* (PPTR), consisting of nine performance factors grouped under three categories: personnel, fiscal, and goals and standards (Ganong, 1981). These two performance measures are shown as Exhibits 2-3 and 2-4.

A multivariate correlational analysis of the data provides these results:

1. highly self-actualizing nurse administrators tolerate ambiguous situations
2. the higher the perceived job stress of these administrators, the lower their perceived performance
3. the more self-actualizing nurse administrators perceive their job stress as lower
4. the level of self-actualizing among these nurse administrators has no significant correlation with their perceived performance.

The findings clearly indicate that the subjects in this study are like self-actualizing people in that they score above the mean in both time competence and inner-directedness on the POI scale.

The multiple regression analysis for the measure of perceived job performance (PPTR) shows the significant contributions of the self-actualizing and tolerance of ambiguity measures to that instrument. This suggests the possible utility of both the POI and the AT-20 measures as predictors of performance for nurse administrators.

The multiple regression analysis for stress shows two strong contributing variables, self-actualizing and age, both at a significant level. These also have significant negative correlations with stress. In view of these findings, and with a significant negative correlation of perceived job stress with perceived job performance, the stress measure appears to be another useful predictor of performance identified by this study. This apparently is the first study that has identified a measurable relationship between job stress and job performance.

These findings may prove useful in considering nurse administrators for promotion from within the hospital or for hiring from outside for that position. Further experience with these measures may well demonstrate their usefulness in the performance evaluation of top administrators in the nursing department or division and thus contribute to the productivity and quality performance of the entire organization.

Exhibit 2-3 Job Stress Indices

		Not at All	Rarely	Some-times	Rather Often	Nearly all the time
Instructions:	For each item listed, circle the number that best describes your answer to the question.					
Question:	How often are you bothered by the following in your work?					
	Job Stress Items					
Stress 1 Responsibility Pressure	1. Feeling you have too much responsibility for the work of others	1	2	3	4	5
	2. Having to do or decide things where mistakes could be quite costly	1	2	3	4	5
	3. Not having enough help or equipment to get the job well done	1	2	3	4	5
Stress 2 Quality Concern	4. Thinking that the *amount* of work you have to do may interfere with how *well* it gets done	1	2	3	4	5
	5. Feeling that you have to do things that are against your better judgment	1	2	3	4	5
	6. Feeling unable to influence your immediate supervisor's decisions and actions that affect you	1	2	3	4	5
Stress 3 Role Conflict	7. Thinking that you'll not be able to meet the conflicting demands of various people you work with	1	2	3	4	5
	8. Not knowing what the people you work with expect of you	1	2	3	4	5
	9. Having to deal with or satisfy too many people	1	2	3	4	5

Exhibit 2-3 continued

	Job Stress Items	Not at All	Rarely	Some-times	Rather Often	Nearly all the time
Stress 4 **Job vs. Non-Job** **Conflict**	10. Feeling that your job tends to interfere with your family life	1	2	3	4	5
	11. Being asked to work overtime when you don't want to	1	2	3	4	5
	12. Feeling trapped in a job you don't like but can't get out of	1	2	3	4	5

		Never	Rarely	Some-times	Fairly Often	Very Often
Stress 5 **Work Load**	13. How often does your job require you to work *very fast?*	1	2	3	4	5
	14. How often does your job require you to work *very hard* (physically or mentally)?	1	2	3	4	5
	15. How often does your job leave you with *little time* to get everything done?	1	2	3	4	5

Source: Reprinted from "A Correlational Study of Relationships Among Self-Actualizing, Tolerance of Ambiguity, Job Stress, and Performance Track Record as perceived by Nurse Administrators" by Joan M. Ganong, Doctoral Dissertation, The Fielding Institute, 1981; *Dissertation Abstracts International, 1981, 42* (11), © 1981, with permission.

Of interest is the fact that the subjects of the study ranged in age from 29 to 64, with a mean of 45.5. As to their educational levels: 20 had earned their diploma in nursing only, 23 had baccalaureate degrees, 40 had earned master's degrees, and one had a doctorate.

The perceived performance track record (Exhibit 2-4) is designed as a self-report questionnaire stimulated in part by Dailey and Madsen (1980). The following descriptive information is from the dissertation (Ganong, 1981).

The questionnaire was developed by me to provide an external criterion measure of this study. It consists of 9 performance

Exhibit 2-4 Perceived Performance Track Record (PPTR)

Purpose:	To elicit a self-report of your performance as a nurse administrator in terms of departmental results under your leadership during the past year.					
Directions:	For each factor listed, circle the number (ranging from 1 as *unsatisfactory* to 5 as *satisfactory*) that best describes how well the nursing department under your leadership has met the standard or norm that you believe is reasonable.					
	Performance Factors	*Self-report based upon your concept of a reasonable criterion for each factor.*				
PPTR 1 **Personnel**	1. Absenteeism	1	2	3	4	5
	2. Turnover	1	2	3	4	5
	3. Patient Care Outcome Audits (or other measure of quality)	1	2	3	4	5
PPTR 2 **Fiscal**	4. Obtains Adequate Budget	1	2	3	4	5
	5. Expenses Stay Within Budget	1	2	3	4	5
	6. Cost/Patient Day (or cost per unit of service)	1	2	3	4	5
PPTR 3 **Goals &** **Standards**	7. Sets Realistic Goals and Measurable Objectives	1	2	3	4	5
	8. Meets Goals and Objectives	1	2	3	4	5
	9. JCAH Evaluation	1	2	3	4	5

Source: Reprinted from "A Correlational Study of Relationships among Self-Actualizing, Tolerance of Ambiguity, Job Stress, and Performance Track Record as Perceived by Nurse Administrators" by Joan M. Ganong, Doctoral Dissertation, The Fielding Institute, 1981; *Dissertation Abstracts International*, 1981, *42*(11), © 1981, with permission.

factors, each to be evaluated as a self-report of performance during the past year in terms of departmental results under each subject's leadership as nurse administrator. The 5-choice scale ranges from 0 to 4, representing a continuum from "not satisfactory" to "satisfactory." The instructions are: "For each factor listed, circle the number which best describes how well the nursing department under your leadership has met the standard or norm which you believe is reasonable."

No other quantitative or qualitative measures of performance can be justified as meaningful because of the wide diversity of circumstances among the hospital population for this study. They vary in terms of ownership and management, philosophy, tradition, adaptation to modern trends, medical staff domination, rural or urban setting, competition for staff, caliber of the chief executive officer, and so on. These and other factors—including length of service of the nurse administrator in a highly volatile job market—significantly influence what can be considered a "reasonable standard or norm." From my personal experience as a nurse administrator, and as consultant/counselor to many hundreds of nurse administrators, I am confident of their being able to use the PPTR for its intended purpose in this study. (p. 124)

There is every reason to believe that these instruments served the research study well. It is to be hoped, however, that others will make further use of both the personality and the performance measures for replication purposes and especially for exploring the practical applications of the findings related to stress and performance track record.

PERFORMANCE APPRAISAL ON THE LINE

The study of the literature by the staff of the Center for Creative Leadership in Greensboro, N.C. (DeVries, Morrison, Shullman, & Gerlach, 1981), noted in Chapter 1, integrates research findings with practical issues gleaned from the appraisal literature, from more than 100 interviews with managers, and survey data from 1,000 managers and professionals. That study focuses on performance appraisal as an organizational intervention. It shows that how a system is put into place and run is as important as which particular system is chosen. It views appraisal as a fundamental process of communication and as one of many management systems in an organization. Specific guidelines are provided on how to select and develop a performance appraisal system and how to conduct an appraisal suited to a given work environment. The authors compare many types of appraisal systems in terms of cost-benefit analysis and weigh the options and trade-offs involved.

The authors ask tough, pragmatic questions that anyone involved with performance appraisal must face, and they attempt to provide answers distilled from their vast research and their own experience. They explain how to gain organizational support for a performance appraisal system; they furnished helpful information on performance appraisal and the law, and discussed many other salient issues. Their prognosis on the changes likely to occur in performance appraisal during the 1980s is well-researched and revealing (DeVries, Morrison, Shullman, & Gerlach, 1981, Jacket). Early in the book the authors review psychometric issues in performance appraisal (PA); discuss validity, reliability, discriminability, and usefulness, then provide a capsule analysis of legal issues in performance measurement (DeVries et al., 1981) as follows:

Legal Issues in Performance Measurement

Before proceeding with a discussion of existing measurement options, it is necessary to examine some of the legal issues of PA. The reason such a discussion follows a description of psychometric issues in a chapter about measurement may not be obvious. In reality, however, the legal guidelines for PA are actually an affirmation of professional principles for sound assessment developed by professionals themselves (American Psychological Association, 1974; Division of Industrial-Organizational Psychology, 1975).

The current [1981] guidelines, in essence, require any test or selection device showing adverse impact to be validated or proved to be related to job performance. This has been, and will continue to be, as much sound psychological and psychometric practice as legal compliance. Yet it seems that it has taken a legal examination of the impact of certain personnel decisions, like PA, to establish consistent standards of practice and stable conceptual frameworks (i.e., PA is a selection device, not just a criterion measure).

The Tower Amendment to the 1964 Civil Rights Act was the first in a continuing series of events to alter the legal context of PA. Specifically, the Tower Amendment approved the use of "professionally developed ability tests" for employment decisions, provided that such tests were not "designed, intended, or used to discriminate because of race, color, religion, sex, or national origin" (Robertson, 1978). EEOC was given legislative responsibility for enforcing this act. In 1966, the EEOC issued guidelines regarding an employer's obligation for testing and selection procedures pertaining to equal employment opportunity. These guidelines were substantially revised in 1970.

In 1971, the Supreme Court handed down a landmark decision in *Griggs v. Duke Power,* incorporating the existing guidelines into a legal framework for employment testing. In essence, the Supreme Court gave legitimacy to guidelines which required that employers produce evidence that selection criteria are related to actual job performance and put the burden of proof on employers to demonstrate nondiscrimination in the presence of adverse impact.

Promotion, retention, and selection decisions were the focus of early court cases involving these guidelines, and PA ratings seemed to serve more as the criteria against which employment decisions were validated rather than being viewed as selection devices or tests themselves (Lazer, 1976). *Brito v. Zia Company* (1973), however, established the applicability of the guidelines to PA ratings as well. In this case, involving layoffs of Spanish-surnamed employees, the court concluded that:

1. Supervisory ratings were vague and subjective measures.
2. The appraisers (supervisors) did not have regular, reasonable, daily contact with employees.
3. Supervisor performance ratings, as selection devices resulting in layoffs, were not scored and administered under appropriately standardized and controlled conditions.

In 1975, the Supreme Court handed down an opinion in *Albemarle Paper Company v. Moody* that upheld the provisions of the extensively revised 1970 guidelines. The court criticized three particular aspects of the testing program:

1. Using subjective supervisory ratings as criteria.
2. Using a test validated only on upper-level positions for entry-level jobs.
3. Validating a test on a group that is not representative of job applicants.

In essence, *Albemarle v. Moody* was the landmark decision that legally required supervisors to use more than vague and subjective criteria in reaching employment decisions and prescribed statistical validation procedures to establish proof of job relatedness.

Washington v. Davis (1976) appeared initially to dilute the growing impact of the EEOC *Guidelines* by refocusing on the need to prove intent to discriminate. The court decided in favor of a police selection procedure that resulted in disproportionate numbers of blacks failing but which showed no intent to discriminate against black applicants. The dilution, however, did not occur. *Washington v. Davis* had been tried under the Constitution (that requires proof of intent) rather than Title VII (which does not). The Title VII framework remained intact and gained momentum through the 1970s.

Also during the 1970s, however, another set of guidelines based on the EEOC model was established by the Office of Federal Contract Compliance. Although similar, these two sets of guidelines differed in the degree of stringency and, in a few cases, actually contradicted each other (Robertson, 1978). The result was that several sets of standards were required for employers instead of just one. Whereas the EEOC still maintained responsibility for enforcement of Title VII legislation, the Civil Service Commission [later renamed the Office of Personnel Management], the Department of Justice, and the Department of Labor also enforced antidiscrimination regulations.

On August 25, 1978, the *Uniform Guidelines on Employee Selection Procedures* were adopted by the four major federal enforcement agencies (EEOC, 1978). These *Guidelines* replaced existing requirements and have provided one consistent set of federal regulations.

The *Guidelines,* building on past regulations, include the following:

1. Employers may not, through the use of any selection device for employment decisions, discriminate against any group protected by Title VII of the Civil Rights Act of 1964 (i.e., on the basis of race, color, religion, sex, or national origin).
2. Employment decisions are any personnel practices that result in selection, training, transfer, retention, or promotion of employees.
3. It is not necessary to establish an *intent* to discriminate to prove discrimination. The presence (or absence) of a disproportionate number from a protected group is defined as prima facie evidence of adverse impact.

The new *Guidelines* include a specific rule of thumb for evaluating adverse impact—the four-fifths, or 80 percent rule. The 80 percent rule states that the selection ratio for protected groups must not fall below 80 percent of the selection ratio for the majority group. In other words, there is a 20 percent buffer zone for selection rate differences; but a difference beyond 20 percent constitutes a prima facie case of adverse impact.

Further, the *Guidelines* do not require validation documentation in all cases—just those cases where the test or selection device (e.g., PA ratings) results in adverse impact on a protected group. For cases in which validation is required, the *Guidelines* recognize content and construct validity as equally acceptable validation options as criterion (empirical) validity evidence.

Also, the *Guidelines* have added the concept of a "bottom-line strategy" to limit the need to validate at each step of any personal selection procedure. The *Guidelines* state that as long as the combined effect of a selection process (e.g., a PA system) does not produce adverse impact, each selection step does not have to be validated separately. In return for this reduction in required validation steps, organizations must now keep records of application and hiring statistics separately by protected group.

Finally, the *Guidelines* appear to be going one step beyond "equal opportunity" by allowing employers to choose alternative selection devices that eliminate adverse impact rather than retaining devices for which differences have been validated. Robertson (1978) views this as a move toward a "concept of equal results."

Several authors have reviewed the *Guidelines* and recent court cases involving PA measures (Cascio & Bernardin [1981]; Holley, Feild, & Barnett, 1976; Odom, 1977). In general, these cases point to the following legal requirements for PA systems:

1. PA ratings should be job related and valid.
2. Job-related performance criteria to be rated should be derived from a thorough job analysis that appropriately represents all significant performance dimensions.
3. PA ratings should be collected under formal standardized conditions.
4. PA ratings should be examined for bias (evidence of adverse impact). Care should be taken—through measurement development, training, and ongoing review—to eliminate bias regarding race, color, sex, religion, and national origin.
5. Organizations should avoid use of supervisory ratings based on vague and subjective factors.

6. PA raters must have personal knowledge and reasonable contact with the job performance to be rated; they must be able to make the appropriate observations.

Thus, from both a psychometric and legal perspective, organizations today do not have the luxury of deciding whether to examine psychometric properties of existing PA programs. The real choice is in selecting among alternative approaches available. (pp. 35–38)

Principal PA Systems in the Literature

DeVries et al.'s first criterion for selecting which existing PA systems to analyze is that the programs should take a stand on the majority of the who, what, when, where, and why questions. These questions relate to such issues as the employee populations covered, whether or not the performance expectations are job relevant, whether the system relates PA events chronologically to other management programs, what the functional relations are to other management programs (strategic planning, compensation, and so forth), and the primary purposes served.

Their second criterion is that some empirical evidence regarding the system's effectiveness should be available.

The third criterion is that at least one actual organizational use of the system should be reported in the literature.

Using these criteria, they reject such approaches as subordinate participation, the performance contingent approach, and the trait-rating scale approach. Table 2-1 shows their evaluation of the cost-effectiveness of the three principal PA systems in the literature. They are summarized as those described as behavior based, such as those with behaviorally anchored rating scales (BARS); those that are effectiveness based, such as the management by objectives (MBO) approach; and the hybrid systems that incorporate the features of several PA approaches and the increased use of MBO. Our results-oriented performance evaluation program (ROPEP) described in Chapters 4 and 5 is essentially such a hybrid system.

DeVries et al. indicate that the hybrid approach is the current vogue in PA. This is at least partially true because a full and accurate picture of job performance requires measuring both behaviors and outcomes. The low rating assigned for organizational acceptance reflects the judgment of the survey authors that managers may perceive that they are being asked to give too much to this process. That may be because the hybrid PA systems have been designed to cover the weaknesses or limits of both the behavior-based and effectiveness-based appraisal systems.

Table 2-1 Cost-Effectiveness of 3 Principal PA Systems in the
              Literature*

	Behavior Based (e.g., BARS)	Effectiveness Based (e.g., MBO)	Hybrid
Costs			
Develop the system (e.g., create the form)	**High**	Low	High
Introduce the system (e.g., train managers)	Moderate	High	High
Maintain the system (e.g., time of managers required; amount of paperwork)	Low	**High**	High
Outcomes			
Chance of fulfilling purposes			
Valid input to administrative decisions (e.g., pay)	**Moderate**	Low	Moderate
Develop employee (e.g., improve performance)	Low	**Moderate**	Moderate
Identify training needs of employees	Moderate	Low	Moderate
Help human resource planning	Low	Low	Moderate
Give legal documentation	**High**	Moderate	High
Organizational acceptance	**Low**	**Moderate**	Low

* Judgments shown in boldface type are those for which the literature provides direct
evidence for the judgment.

Source: Reprinted from *Performance Appraised on the Line* by D.L. DeVries, A.M. Morrison, S.L.
Shullman, and M.L. Gerlach with permission of John Wiley & Sons, Inc., © 1981.

Whereas BARS appears to be particularly responsive to administrative
uses and MBO seems most appropriate for developing employees, the
hybrid attempts to achieve both. Nurse managers should find it to be a
productive exercise to evaluate their own PA system using the factors in
Exhibit 2-2. This may be especially fruitful if they have been involved in
the development, revision, and/or continuing use of their current PA system.

What System Works Best?

The summing up by DeVries et al. of their analyses recalls some of Beaulieu's comments earlier in this chapter. DeVries et al. conclude:

> If the overriding question . . . is "What works?" then the answer is "We don't know." We do know what does not work. Traditional trait-oriented graphic-rating scales may be easy to implement, but what they give you is not likely to stand up to any tests—particularly those a court of law is likely to apply.
>
> In principle, the hybrid system appears to cover best all the bases. It should be useful both in helping make administrative decisions and for giving the employee useful feedback. Five years from now we should be in a better position to judge the impact of hybrid systems. A hybrid system should be treated as a second- or third-generation PA system. It is unlikely to work in an organization with no prior PA program or in an organization recently "burned" by PA (i.e., asked to invest much in PA with little return).
>
> But what does it mean "to work?" Some of the most difficult work in reassessing existing or creating new PA systems is in identifying a finite set of goals for the system. Until you do so, making changes in the mechanics of the system can be a random act. Defining and limiting the goals of PA are so difficult because PA involves multiple constituencies both in and outside the organization. . . .
>
> Successful PA is an ephemeral experience. Even in organizations in which PA is being done regularly and competently by managers there still seems to be a top management that remains unconcerned about the merit of its procedure. The reason may reside in the list of outcomes typically assigned to PA [Table 2-1]. PA is asked to serve other human resource programs. Even if PA does serve these other programs successfully, it is a step away from the more primary goal of a more efficient and humane use of the human resources in the organization.
>
> Measuring this latter goal requires translating human resources into financial terms. Employees can be viewed as significant assets in organizations, assets that should be capitalized on. Dahl (1979) and others are developing human resource accounting models that will give organizations more tangible goals for their

human resource programs. The value of translating human resource programs into financial impact can be seen in the Mirvis and Lawler (1977) study of attitude surveys. Applying such accounting procedures is a much-needed and promising redefinition of the goals of such human resource programs as PA. (pp. 91–93)

Defining PA in the 1980s

DeVries et al. summarize the expected impact upon the purposes of PA and supplemental programs during the 1980s of such factors as government regulation, economic conditions, labor characteristics, and employee participation:

- PA, when considered as a specific, annual event, will have as its primary purpose the documentation of administrative decisions for legal protection.
- PA will be used for human resource planning or as appraisal documents, to assess the needs and availability of such resources to carry out the organization's goals.
- PA will be used to meet the demands of members of the work force for participation in decisions that affect their own jobs and their own lives.

DeVries et al. say that increased productivity is certain to be a goal of PA for many organizations in the years ahead. Yet they point out that Yankelovich (1979) suggests that true productivity depends ultimately on intangibles such as dedication, caring, and a sense of responsibility for giving real service. This commentary has particular significance in health care organizations.

DeVries et al. also believe that formal PA ratings are likely to be supplemented with individualized objectives for which some demonstrable measures of success can be devised. However, they say, the issue of subjectivity still remains. The criterion standards by which many workers judge themselves and their jobs are largely subjective. But DeVries et al. expect subjectivity in managerial judgment of worker performance to be less of a problem if managers come to understand the value orientation of this new breed of employees. They cite Ford (1979): "If we involve these people in our planning, if we respect them for their values and attitudes, if we get to know them as individuals, then . . . we will have greater productivity than less, and more harmony then acrimony."

Managers on the Firing Line

DeVries et al. (1981) provide the following conclusion:

> Although historically the manager-subordinate relationship has been one in which the manager could set the rules and which was characterized by some privacy, that is changing. Managers must realize that how they handle key decisions such as promotion and termination is of interest to several parties, including one or more federal regulatory agencies. You need to prepare and regularly reinforce managers in strategies for handling employees in ways that capitalize on the more complex needs they now bring to the job. Clearly, managerial development will need to move from a once-in-a-lifetime "laying down the rules" toward an annual updating and expanding of skills.
>
> *PA—deciding what it is and is not.* One theme [of] this review . . . was the unrealistic number of responsibilities some organizations assign PA. Those responsibilities will be even greater in the 1980s. The challenge will be to build new programs around such themes as career development and job enrichment that have their own separate identity and are not assigned to the PA agenda. That agenda is already chock full of significant issues. (p. 139)

This book, the most comprehensive overview of performance appraisal to date, is particularly pertinent for nurse managers (and hospital personnel departments) who are, or plan to be, involved in revising and updating their current appraisal program. While it may not be necessary to try to become an expert in all of the design features that are important to performance appraisal, at the very least it is essential to be aware of the complexities and stumbling blocks that must be faced.

DILEMMAS IN SALARY COMPRESSION, MERIT PAY

Dilemma is defined as a choice between two equal alternatives. Dilemmas in performance appraisal are discussed by at least two other sources referred to in this book (DeVries et al., 1981; Low, 1976, in Chapter 3, infra). Another survey report, *Paying for Performance and Position* (Steele, 1982), presents dilemmas in salary compression and merit pay being experienced by organizations generally throughout the country. It is significant here because so many organizations, including hospitals, use performance appraisal for decisions affecting salary adjustments, merit increases, and promotion.

The findings are based on analysis of data from 613 organizations representing a wide cross-section of American industry. Of these, 9.1 percent are medical/health care/nonprofit organizations. Of all responding organizations, 67 percent indicated that they were struggling with the problem of salary compression—the narrowing of the gap between managers' salaries and what their highest paid hourly personnel received. In all, 68 percent of medical/health service organizations reporting cited this problem.

Steele (1982) brings the problem into focus in his first two paragraphs:

> Most managers have come to expect periodic merit increases as the just rewards for jobs well done—for contributing successfully to organizational objectives. And virtually all salary administration policies are founded on the concept that meritorious performance should be rewarded and that higher levels of compensation should go to those who apply specialized skills or supervise the work of others.

> But there's a problem. For almost a decade, many managers have been watching the compensation gap between themselves and their subordinates become narrower and narrower. And in extreme cases, when the hourly workers' overtime pay is added on, the worker receives a larger paycheck than the supervisor. At the same time, merit increases have simply not kept up with inflation. Since 1973, the average manager has "lost" more than 10 percent in buying power. Indeed, the combined problems of salary compression and the inability to properly reward meritorious performance have created one of the most difficult periods in the area of compensation administration that many organizations have had to deal with. (p. 7)

In the late seventies, while helping a client update a hospitalwide performance appraisal program, the authors were asked about installation of a merit rating system. Their response: "Don't do it." The industrial relations director of the hospital commented, "That's interesting. That is exactly what two other consultants have told us recently."

The reason for the authors' stance on merit rating has to do with the wide variety of factors that, from a practical standpoint, influence the actual wages and salaries paid to individuals (enumerated in Chapter 1). And Steele reports:

Merit systems are floundering. For some organizations, the approach to merit pay has become so entrenched in rigid formulae, and so diluted by other considerations (an employee's length of service, for example) that it reflects "merit" in name only. Furthermore, problems with the performance appraisal system—the process of determining who is doing an above-adequate job and who isn't—frequently pull the carpet out from under otherwise sound merit administration systems. Newer forms of organizational structure (matrix arrangements, for example) add additional complications, as does company size. And, of course, an organization's ability to pay—in other words, its profitability—can dampen pay-for-performance programs considerably. (p. 18)

Table 2-2 presents the respondents' degree of support for a variety of possible solutions to salary administration problems. Solution #11, eliminating the merit system in favor of a general increase and bonus program, received the least support of all (85 percent of the sample rejected it). This is not surprising, considering the influence of inertia and conventional thinking. But bonus and incentive programs are a topic for discussion in hospital board rooms. Yet, the concept of "add-on" bonuses for performance has not really caught on in health care institutions except in investor-owned hospitals. They are well ahead of all others in paying incentives (Cole, 1982, p. 82).

Steele's report concludes with speculation:

Perhaps there are no broadly viable or practical solutions, especially to the merit increase/inflation problem. Perhaps many organizations will continue to watch helplessly as their employees' real income erodes further and further, the result of continued high levels of inflation. Or perhaps this problem, too, will simply go away in time.

If the problem doesn't go away, and inflation again escalates to the painfully high levels that marked the 1970s, we can expect increased restraints on merit budgets. Further compression may well occur between supervisors' earnings and their hourly and college-graduate subordinates. In this case, the present survey data represent a kind of snapshot: one frozen moment in the inexorable dawning of the age of egalitarianism. (p. 50)

This report deserves close attention by nurse administrators and hospital personnel directors. It can be particularly useful during the planning stages

Table 2-2 Support for Solutions to Salary Administration Problems

Solutions	Organizations with Compression (%)		Organizations without Compression (%)	
	No Support	Moderate to Strong Support	No Support	Moderate to Strong Support
1. Grant periodic increases for all salaried classifications	47.7	48.0	56.3*	35.3*
2. Grant general increases for affected job classes only	45.0	49.9	47.4	42.1*
3. Establish or broaden profit sharing to include all salaried supervision	40.1	47.9	33.7*	49.5
4. Institute (or broaden current) program to promote college relations and enhance recruiting success	20.4	69.4	26.8*	58.9*
5. Forgo recruiting at more prestigious schools	53.1	35.0	51.6	28.4*
6. Recruit candidates of lesser academic standing	68.1	23.1	64.2	19.5
7. Develop or expand in-house skill training, especially in high-demand skill areas	5.0	70.9	5.1	76.6
8. Expand use of contract houses, consultants to supplement work force in high-demand skill areas	45.3	49.6	42.1	47.4
9. Create fewer job classifications and broaden their rate ranges	65.0	30.4	60.0	29.5
10. Establish or use a bonus program that instantly rewards good performance or special effort	28.2	67.4	30.5	60.0*
11. Eliminate merit system in favor of a general increase and bonus program	85.2	11.4	82.1	10.0
12. Adopt harder line in union negotiations to hold down size of wage increases	13.9	54.5	17.9	39.5*
13. Modify or eliminate COLA clauses	20.0	46.0	23.7	36.8*

Table 2-2 continued

	Organizations with Compression (%)		Organizations without Compression (%)	
Solutions	No Support	Moderate to Strong Support	No Support	Moderate to Strong Support
14. Negotiate (or establish) fewer wage levels among hourly unit employees	44.3	36.0	37.9	33.7
15. Grant additional compensation for overtime hours worked to:				
First- and second-line supervisors	20.7	70.6*	35.3*	50.5*
All supervisors up to middle management	42.1	47.7*	49.5*	34.8*

* The difference between the percentages is statistically significant at the .05 level or better.

Source: Reprinted from *Paying for Performance and Position: Dilemmas in Salary Compression and Merit Pay,* AMA Survey Report, by J.S. Steele, with permission of American Management Associations, © 1982, p. 45.

---

when a performance appraisal program is being reviewed and updated. It also can be helpful in connection with planning the details of a career ladder program so that it is carefully integrated with the performance appraisal criteria and the wage and salary administration program.

For Discussion Purposes

As your performance appraisal task force continues its work, you begin to explore the literature on the subject more widely. Some of the research findings and other studies begin to raise some questions in your mind about the legal aspects of performance appraisal, merit rating, wage administration, and related dilemmas. For example, one item you find is this:

Watch for more employees contending that personnel policies— even implied or unwritten ones—are enforceable employment contracts—consultant Harry Levinson recommends identifying these psychological contracts in some detail, including what's expected on both sides (also recording all incidents, performance appraisals, etc. to support dismissals). (Kennedy, 1983)

As a result, you begin to question some of the initial assumptions you adopted, consciously or not, in stating the purposes for your appraisal program. You ask yourselves:

1. Should performance appraisal serve the same purposes as merit rating?
2. Should performance reviews be directly related to wage and salary decisions?
3. Does our appraisal plan conform to legal requirements?
4. Can (and should) we use the same plan for nurse managers as well as other nursing department employees?
5. Does our plan facilitate the use of in-house career ladders?

These and similar questions cause you to rethink the purposes you have been developing and lead you into some broader concerns than you had anticipated. In addition, you begin to see more clearly the implications of the design and techniques of the performance appraisal program itself.

Describe the dilemmas you face.

NOTES

American Psychological Association & National Council on Measurement in Education. *Standards for educational tests*. Washington, D.C.: American Psychological Association, 1974.

Beaulieu, R. An easier look at performance appraisal. *Training and Development Journal,* October 1980, *34*(10), 56–58.

Cascio, W.F., & Bernardin, H.J. Implications of performance appraisal litigation for personnel decisions. *Personnel Psychology,* 1981, *34*(2), 211–236.

Cole, B.S. Top hospital managers win 11.4% salary increase. *Modern Healthcare,* December 1982, *12*(12).

Dahl, H.L., Jr. Meauring the ROI. *Management Review,* January 1979, *68*(1), 44–50.

Dailey, C. *Using the track record approach*. New York: AMACOM, 1982.

Dailey, C., & Madsen, A. *How to evaluate people in business*. New York: McGraw-Hill Book Company, 1980.

DeVries, D.L.; Morrison, A.M.; Shullman, S.L.; & Gerlach, M.L. *Performance appraisal on the line*. New York: John Wiley & Sons, Inc., 1981.

Division of Industrial-Organizational Psychology. *Principles for the validation and use of personnel selection procedures*. Dayton, Ohio: American Psychological Association, 1975.

Equal Employment Opportunity Commission. Uniform guidelines on employee selection procedures. *Federal Register,* August 25, 1978, *43*(166), 38290–38309.

Ford, T.M. Tomorrow's employee: The supervisor's greatest challenge. *Supervisory Management,* 1979, *24*(6), 9–11.

Ganong, J.M. A. correlational study of relationships among self-actualizing, tolerance of ambiguity, job stress, and performance track record as perceived by nurse administrators. (Doctoral dissertation, The Fielding Institute, 1981). *Dissertation Abstracts International,* 1981, *42*(11), (University Microfilms No. DA8207884).

Ganong, J.M., & Ganong, W.L. ABP for nursing administration. *Journal of Nursing Administration,* May–June 1973. *3*(3), 6.

Ganong, J.M., & Ganong, W.L. *HELP with annual budgetary planning and control.* Chapel Hill, N.C.: W.L. Ganong Co., 1976.

Ganong, W.L. & Ganong, J.M. *The G-GRAM: Newsletter for Nurse Managers and Educators,* November 1981, *8*(6), Special Report.

Ganong, W.L., & Ganong, J.M. *The G-GRAM: Newsletter for Nurse Managers and Educators,* 1982, *9*(2).

Gilbert, T. *Human competence: Engineering worthy performance.* New York: McGraw-Hill Book Company, 1978.

Holley, W.H., Feild, H.S., & Barnett, N.J. Analyzing performance appraisal systems. *Personnel Journal,* 1976, *55,* 457–463.

House, J.; Wells, J.; Landerman, L.; McMichael, A.; & Kaplan, B. Occupational stress and health among workers. *Journal of Health and Social Behavior,* 1979, *20,* 139–160.

Kennedy, J. Newsletter comment. *Consultant's News,* April 1983.

Lazer, R.I. The discrimination danger in performance appraisal. *The Conference Board Record,* March 1976, 60–64.

Low, A. *Zen and creative management.* Garden City, N.Y.: Anchor Press/Doubleday, 1976.

MacDonald, A. Revised scale for ambiguity tolerance: Reliability and validity. *Psychological Reports,* 1970, *26,* 791–798.

McGregor, D. An uneasy look at performance appraisal. *Harvard Business Review,* May/June 1957, *22*(3), 133–138.

Mintzberg, H. The nature of managerial work. New York: Harper & Row, Publishers, Inc., 1973.

Mirvis, P.J., & Lawler, E.E., III. Measuring the financial impact of employee attitudes. *Journal of Applied Psychology,* 1977, *62,* 1–8.

Odom, J.V. *Performance appraisal: Legal aspects* (Tech. Rep. No. 3). Greensboro, N.C.: Center for Creative Leadership, May 1977.

Robertson, D.E. New directions in EEO guidelines. *Personnel Journal,* 1978, *57,* 360–363; 394.

Shostrom, E.L. A test for the measurement of self-actualization. *Education and Psychological Measurement,* 1964, *24,* 207–218.

Shostrom, E.L. *Man, the manipulator.* New York: Bantam Books, Inc., 1968.

Steele, J.W. *Paying for performance and position: Dilemmas in salary compression and merit pay.* New York: American Management Associations, 1982.

Yankelovich, D. Yankelovich on today's workers: We need new motivational tools. *Industry Week,* August 6, 1979, *202*(3), 61–65, 68.

Chapter 3

Organizing for Performance Appraisal

HEALTH CARE CONCEPTS IN A CHANGING SOCIETY

This chapter provides an orderly approach to introducing a new performance appraisal plan or modifying one that exists already. Each organization and department must begin from where it is now with performance appraisal and other factors that affect such a plan. Some of these factors are specific to the nursing department itself, others are organizationwide. Still others are nationwide, influencing the trends and climate in the health care industry as a whole.

Nurse managers should be aware of these factors and their direct or indirect influence on attempts to implement effective performance appraisal as part of their responsibilities for productivity.

The demands of day-to-day operational management on every nurse manager occur in the broad framework of a dynamic, free-wheeling, ever-changing internal and external environment. These environmental factors are presented in Table 3-1. An understanding of these concepts may help nurse managers in discharging their role as managers of change and in handling the attendant problems and conflicts. At the very least, consideration of these concepts may help to develop a philosophical outlook and provide a sound perspective for managing in an effective active way rather than simply reacting to events and trends.

Table 3-1 conveys the kaleidoscopic pattern, the future shock (Toffler, 1974), of multitudinous changes in the health care environment. This is done within the framework of the groups affected by (and effecting) the changes from Concept A to Concept B. Concept A embraces the historical and conventional attributes and practices characteristic of older generations. Concept B is represented by the current and innovative attributes and practices of persons moving with the times, with an up-to-date and forward-looking orientation and motivation.

Table 3-1 Panorama of Health Care Concepts in a Rapidly Changing Society

Concepts	Groups Affected by (and Effecting) Change								
	Nursing	Medicine	Management	Hospitals	Trustees	Consumers	Government	JCAH	Public Health
A*	Tasks and Routines	Diagnose Rx Cure	Authoritarian	Single Units	Fund Raising	Passive	Increasing Rules and Regulations	Higher Standards	Prevention
A/B	The ABies: Caught in the middle; or using the best of both concepts; or moving toward Concept B.								
B**	The Nursing Process	+ Care Prevention Share	Participative	Multi-Hospital Systems + Competition	+ Responsibility for Q. A.	Active	Changing R & R: Increasing Competition, TEFRA/PPS	Changing Standards	Prevention +

* CONCEPT A: Historical/Conventional Attributes
** CONCEPT B: Current/Innovative Attributes

Source: Reprinted from *G-Gram newsletter for nurse managers and educators* by Joan M. Ganong and Warren L. Ganong. Chapel Hill, N.C.: W.L. Ganong Co., March/April 1983, *10*(2), 3.

These two concepts are highlighted by a single characteristic for each group as an indication of the flow from *then* to *now*. These elements were selected from among many existing in a wide variety of settings across the country.

Thus nursing has shifted from a task-and-routine orientation (Concept A) to the use of the nursing process for improved individual care based on patients' individual needs and goals (Concept B). For medicine, Concept A is presented as the traditional diagnosis/prescription/cure emphasis while Concept B continues that emphasis but with enlightened attention to holistic care with more attention to maintaining health, prevention of disease, and increased responsibility by patients in medical care decisions (signified by the + in the table).

The trend in enlightened management clearly is from Concept A (authoritarian) to Concept B (participative). The trend in hospital ownership and operation is away from individual, free-standing, community-owned institutions (Concept A) to multihospital systems with some form of centralized ownership and control and varying degrees of decentralized management and competition (+ in the table, Concept B). By 1985 half of all hospitals will be part of multihospital groups.

Consumers used to be characterized by their passive submission to doctors and nurses (Concept A). Now both consumers and employees tend toward activism, with more direct involvement in decisions affecting their care as patients and their working conditions as employees (Concept B). So it is with the other groups and elements in the chart.

The ABies, of course, are those shown as somewhere in the middle range between Concepts A and B because of their own individual proclivities or because of the nature of their internal/external workworld environments. These are people who may feel caught in the middle, or they may be using the best of both concepts as appropriate in their own situations, or they may feel that they are moving strongly toward Concept B but have not yet overcome some of the roadblocks in their path.

Nurse managers may add attributes or characteristics that seem to fit either concept designation for the groups affected by, and effecting, changes in their own personal workworld. Discussion of these factors with others can help clarify the big picture within which nurse managers now function, attempting to maintain or improve productivity with such management techniques as performance appraisal.

"When in doubt, read the instructions." Good advice. A successful entrepreneur in New England, when asked how he did it, said, "I read the book and did what it said to do." That explains it in words of one syllable. An oversimplification perhaps, but there certainly is merit in reading the books and following the instructions. This leads from the broad considerations of health care concepts to a more specific step in organizing for performance appraisal for productivity: completing the nursing organization inventory checklist (Table 3-2).

NURSING ORGANIZATION INVENTORY CHECKLIST

This checklist is a guide to taking stock of a significant number of interrelated organizational elements that affect performance appraisal as a vital technique in a human resources management program. Most of the items are likely to be available now in one form or another. Some will require updating. All are important.

Even if some prove to be only peripherally significant in connection with performance appraisal, the review process offers fringe benefits for those involved. Participation provides a valuable self-development experience with tangible spin-off results in connection with other programs and objectives. For nurse managers, this can become a helpful learning opportunity in conceptualizing the interdependence of the management functions, techniques, and skills in achieving patient care goals.

Completion of the nursing organization inventory checklist can be assigned to a special task force of several members of the nursing management group. At the outset, it is necessary to identify others in the nursing department and in administration who can serve as resources in exploring the inventory items.

The following item-by-item commentary on Table 3-2 suggests what to look for and how to evaluate each factor in terms of its relevance to both performance appraisal and a career ladder program.

1. Hospital Organization Chart

The nurse manager should see the hospital organizational manual for a copy of the organization chart or obtain a copy from the report of the hospital administrator submitted to the visitation team at the last inspection by the Joint Commission for the Accreditation of Hospitals (JCAH). It should be available from the hospital administrator's or the nursing office.

2. Nursing Organization Chart

If not available on each unit, a copy should be obtained from the nursing administrator's office. Is it clear? Who has 24-hour responsibility for each unit? Who is "boss" to each person on evenings and nights? Who evaluates each person's performance and recommends that individual's pay scale?

Table 3-2 Nursing Organization Inventory Checklist

An Audit of Where We Are Now in Our Departmental Workworld

Prepared by _____ Title _____ Date _____

Instructions: See accompanying description of each item. Use this checklist to indicate availability and adequacy of each item, and whatever follow-through you decide is required. (Substitute your health care agency name for "hospitals" in the item list.)

Item	Available?		Reviewed	Understandable?		Follow Through
	Yes	No (when?)	(date)	OK	Not OK	(What? Who? When?)
1. Hospital Organization Chart						
2. Nursing Organization Chart						
3. Support Personnel:						
Systems & Planning Coordinator						
Staffing & Budget Coordinator						
Nurse Recruiting Coordinator						
Unit Instructors						
Clinical Specialists						
Quality Assurance Coordinator						
4. Hospital Policy Manual						
5. Nursing Policy Manual						
6. Hospital Goals & Objectives						
7. Nursing Goals & Objectives						
8. Hospital Budget(s)						
9. Nursing Budget(s)						
10. Wage and Salary Scales						
11. Job Descriptions						
12. Performance Descriptions						

Table 3-2 continued

Item	Available? Yes	No (when?)	Reviewed (date)	Understandable? OK	Not OK	Follow Through (What? Who? When?)
13. Performance Evaluation Plan						
14. Labor Union Contract						
15. Employee Handbook						
16. Workworld of Nurse Mgr.:						
Values						
Motivation						
Knowledge						
Skills						
Clinical Management						
Operational Management						
Nurse Manager as Hospital Integrator						
Unit Profile						
17. Nursing Modalities Defined						
18. Nursing Roles Defined						
19. Recruitment						
20. Orientation						
21. Staff Development						
22. Staffing						
23. Other:						

Source: Reprinted from HELP with Career Ladders in Nursing by Joan M. Ganong and Warren L. Ganong with permission of W.L. Ganong Co., © 1982, p. 16.

Does the chart help to answer these questions? Should it? Who will help each person get additional training on the job or prepare the person for advancement?

3. Support Personnel

Are specific positions shown on the nursing organization chart (or are other provisions made) for persons who are qualified to give technical and staff assistance to nurse managers at all levels with:

- quality assurance
- improving systems and procedures
- cost containment
- developing cyclical (or other) staffing schedules
- program planning (as basis for budgeting)
- budgetary planning, interpretation, and coordination
- recruitment of qualified nursing personnel
- continuing orientation and clinical instruction at the unit level
- specialized high-level clinical nursing expertise?

Have the head nurse and other nurse managers been oriented to the effective use of such support personnel? How much of such support can be provided by administrative staff persons or by other nurse managers or supervisors? How these questions are answered affects the nurse managers' cost-containment efforts, employee care plans, and job progression opportunities.

4. Hospital Policy Manual

This manual should be examined to determine administration's orientation and attitude toward people, both patients and employees. It should contain a statement of philosophy, beliefs, or guidelines related to human resources management. Every reference to the organization's responsibility for employee welfare and opportunity should be identified. Performance appraisal and career ladders can succeed only if there is a suitable philosophical base, as well as economically sound motivation, for such an organizational effort.

5. Nursing Policy Manual

The statements of nursing philosophy and objectives need review to assure that they are consistent with those of the hospital. They should provide a clear, firm base for a career ladder program.

6. Hospital Goals and Objectives

The nurse manager should have a copy of these for this year. What about next year's? Do the hospital's and department's current goals and objectives reflect the policy manual content? How did nursing contribute to defining these goals and objectives? If nursing had inadequate opportunity to contribute, the manager should take the necessary steps to become more involved in planning next year's (and subsequent years') goals and objectives. This is vital, since nursing must support the hospital goals and objectives.

7. Nursing Goals and Objectives

These necessarily reflect the hospital goals and objectives as well as the contributions of all the nursing unit management personnel. Are these goals and objectives available on each patient care unit? Has each unit developed its own for the current year? Next year? Are these clearly related to the unit patient care program? To what extent did the medical staff on each service contribute to such program planning? Such planning is essential as a basis for preparing (and, later, controlling) next year's budget.

8. Hospital Budget(s)

Nursing accounts for approximately 40 percent of the operating budget of the typical general hospital. When the capital budget is included, that proportion rises to upward of 70 percent of the budget. Thus nursing has a major concern with the hospital budget. Is it available to the nurse managers in its entirety?

An informative exercise is to add to the hospital organization chart the total annual operating budget figures beside the name of each department head. What does it indicate about the interdepartmental relationships and relative fiscal responsibility of other department heads compared with head nurses and other nurse managers? What influence is a career ladder program in nursing, with updated performance appraisal, likely to have on the hospital budget? To what extent should this question be considered in nursing department planning? (It may well help to reduce expenses.)

9. Nursing Budget(s)

Every nurse at all levels must be involved with budgetary planning and control. A financial organization chart should be set up in nursing (as in the hospital budget) as a starting point. Points to consider are (1) who has managerial responsibility for each portion of the budget? (2) Who actually spends (uses up) each of the dollars in the operating budget? (3) What is the impact of other items in this checklist on the size of the operating budget? How will a career ladder program affect the budget—short term, long term? All nurse managers need to be familiar enough with budget matters to discuss the foregoing informatively.

10. Wage and Salary Scales

Are these available to all the nurse managers? Do they understand how these scales were established? The management technique used to establish the relative worth of jobs is called job and salary evaluation. Does the hospital use such a method? How recently were wage and salary scales reviewed and updated? Is individual performance considered in determining the specific wage rate for a person? Merit rating (or employee evaluation) is the management technique sometimes used to help determine each person's wage within the rate range for a particular job classification.

11. Job Descriptions

Are these available to every employee? When were they last reviewed and updated? Job descriptions serve as the basis for job and salary evaluation and hence influence decisions regarding the compensation scales.

12. Performance Descriptions

These are different from job descriptions. A performance description is a statement of the *purpose* of a job, the major performance responsibilities (grouped by persons *to whom* the responsibilities exist), and *measures* of satisfactory performance. It is prepared by a process of performance analysis by employees with their own managers (supervisors, department heads, bosses). Its purpose is to reach agreement and understanding, between employee and manager, regarding the former's performance responsibilities so that meaningful, continuing self-evaluation of performance can take place. The emphasis in preparation of a performance description is in reaching a mutual understanding regarding who is to do what for whom, when, and how well so there can be later agreement as to what actually was done for whom, when, and how well.

13. Performance Evaluation Plan

Performance evaluation is the measurement of the results of a person's work effort compared with previously agreed upon standards. This is different from the typical merit rating and employee appraisal plans used in hospitals. The "measures of satisfactory performance" (for the various performance responsibilities identified in the performance description) are used as the basis for evaluation. Such a simple result-oriented performance evaluation program (ROPEP, discussed in detail in Chapters 4 et seq.) becomes a key management technique for making decisions on wages and salaries, promotions, and training. Thus it is a most useful component of a career ladder program.

14. Labor Union Contract

Whenever any group of employees are members of a bargaining unit, planning for performance appraisal and a career ladder program is more complicated. Since a career ladder affects a number of factors involving conditions of employment, it may well become a matter for collective bargaining. This need not necessarily pose any problems but it is something that has to be part of planning. As a matter of fact, when representatives of the bargaining unit are included from the beginning in planning for career ladders, the program can become a major asset at the bargaining table.

15. Employee Handbook

An employee handbook is valuable for every hospital whether or not some employee groups are members of a bargaining unit. The handbook is an important orientation tool for new employees and a continuing source of pertinent information for all. The best handbooks are designed to permit continual updating so that correct current information always is available. For those who are members of a union, the handbook is an important supplement to the union contract. The handbook (and the contract) should contain a description of the career ladder program.

16. Workworld of the Nurse Manager

Figure 3-1 is a graphic presentation of you at the center of your work-world. It applies to you as a staff nurse, head nurse, or nurse manager at any level. The key components of you and your apperceptive mass (depicted as your left brain/right brain) are your values, motivation, knowledge and

Figure 3-1 My Workworld

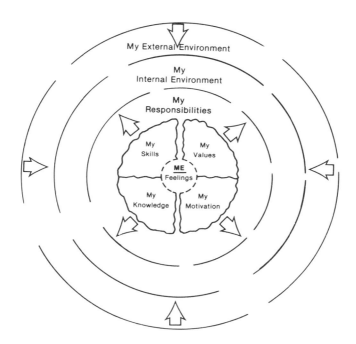

Source: Evolved from *HELP for the Head Nurse* (4th ed.) by Joan M. Ganong and Warren L. Ganong with permission of W.L. Ganong Co., © 1981.

skills. Each of these components influences your reactions to what happens around you, the manner in which you resolve problems, the quality of your decision making and the way in which you carry out your responsibilities. Your responsibilities (the next circular area beyond yourself) include your three major performance areas: patient care management, human resources management, and operational management. These responsibilities are carried out within your hospital (your "internal environment") comprised of hospital administration, the medical staff, and all of the other departments and supportive services of your health care agency.

You and your hospital exist in a community, state and federal environment composed of many elements—your "external environment" of the outer circle. All of these external elements have a significant influence on your hospital and how it is operated. These diverse environmental factors also influence, directly and indirectly (consciously and subconsciously), the decisions you must make in your own job. The higher the level of your management job, the greater the influence of the environmental factors on your own personal workworld—shown by the inward-pointing arrows in the figure.

The outward-pointing arrows show your influence upon the persons in your internal/external environments. You can affect your workworld more than you may realize. Some of the concepts of Figure 3-1 parallel Kurt Lewin's field theory (Lewin, 1951). As Meissner (1978) says, Lewin's field approach has influenced greatly the study of group and social processes.

> The fundamental concept in Lewin's system is the 'life space,' the sum of all facts that determine the person's behavior at a given point in time. The life space includes two primary dimensions: the psychological environment and the person himself. The psychological environment is the external or physical environment, insofar as it determines the person's behavior. . . . The second dimension of the life space in Lewin's analysis is the person. The person's motivation comes from need states. The need system is in a state of tension or 'hunger' (p. 136).

Thus the model of you at the center of your workworld helps with understanding how the impact of internal and external forces affects your behavior as goal-directed action.

Nurse managers are most effective in a hospital setting when they become successful hospital integrators. This means that they develop the skills to coordinate on their units the services rendered to patients and the unit by other hospital departments. This integrating role must be exercised even though these other departments and services are not part of the nursing budget. The day may come, however, when each nurse manager will receive a monthly statement showing the expenses of services by other entities performed on behalf of the patients on the unit (or other segment of the nursing department).

The patient unit profile is the detailed definition of each unit's patient population, the kind of care provided, employee care plans, patterns of interdepartmental relations, physical facilities, special resources, and similar factors that make this entity unique. The profile thus, is a written description of a special segment of the nursing department organization. Every member of the unit can contribute to preparing such a profile. Such an experience is useful because it can help strengthen the sense of organizational unity and builds morale among personnel on all three shifts.

17. Nursing Modality Defined

What patient care modalities are in use? These are so important that they deserve separate consideration. They influence everything else—from the structure of the nursing organization to the orientation and training of personnel and the day-to-day components of every person's performance. Many departments are introducing primary nursing, a process-oriented nursing system, or some other variation of their more traditional team or functional nursing. In fact, most nursing departments tend to be in a state of transition rather than remaining static in their care programs. Introduction of career ladders need not be deferred for these reasons. But it is important that there be a clearly defined direction for the developing patient care programs and nursing care modalities so that these can be taken into account in planning career ladders.

18. Nursing Roles Defined

The proliferation of new job titles, new organizational patterns, and changing concepts of health care services generally is continuing to cause frustration and confusion among nursing personnel. This is understandable. A review of all of the previous items in the inventory checklist may suggest that their adequate evaluation and further implementation will lead logically to better definition of the roles of all nursing personnel. This is true. In addition, the steps involved in introducing a career ladder as a management technique will help provide a better understanding and sharper definition of the performance requirements for every position on all four career tracks—clinical, educational, management, and research.

19. Recruitment

What is the recruitment program for nursing personnel? How successful is it? To ensure optimum results, summarize and describe in detail all aspects of the recruitment efforts, including qualitative and quantitative data to show cost/benefit comparisons.

Recruitment of nursing personnel will affect, and be affected by, the introduction of career ladders. Involvement of present personnel in planning and implementing such ladders tends to reduce turnover. As each step in the program is carried out, interpersonal relations at all levels should improve. Staff members achieve a better understanding of their performance responsibilities and how they can move ahead if they wish to do so.

Once the word gets around among recruitment sources that a career ladder program is in operation, it will be easier to attract the desired kinds of applicants. This fact should be used in recruitment literature and in recruiting contacts during the early stages of the program's implementation. This will help focus attention on an important benefit of a career ladder and may influence the ultimate design of the program itself.

20. Orientation

What is the caliber of the orientation program? How well is each new employee's orientation to the job tailored to that person's specific needs? Such orientation is, after all, the first and fateful beginning of each employee's career with the manager and agency. Does the kind of orientation provided adequately set the tone for the manager's concept of a career ladder and performance appraisal? Should orientation efforts be improved before a career ladder is started?

21. Staff Development

How is the staff development program, including inservice and continuing education, organized now? The persons in these activities will need to be deeply involved with career ladder planning. They can contribute much to the development of the criteria and training programs that define levels and the qualifying procedures, working in close cooperation with the nurse managers and practitioners.

22. Staffing

Is this considered a continuing problem by managers and staff? Or is staffing viewed as simply another necessary but manageable chore? The nurse manager's perception of the staffing situation affects how it is handled. Much can be done about unit-specific staffing when it is considered in relation to the nursing care modality, organizational structure, unit cluster decentralization, unit geography, personnel policies, budget, and recruitment program (Deines, 1983). Suitable performance appraisal and career ladder programs can contribute to better staffing but will achieve a high degree of cost effectiveness only in conjunction with an orderly review of all the other factors that influence the staffing picture.

23. Other

Other items can be added to the checklist as the nurse manager considers them significant in completing the nursing organization inventory.

NURSING ORGANIZATION INVENTORY AS MANAGEMENT AUDIT

It is important to keep in mind that the purpose in using the nursing organization inventory checklist is to facilitate implementation or revision of the performance appraisal program as an essential component of human resources management and career ladder administration. This requires focusing clearly on the objectives of performance appraisal in the nursing department (see Chapter 1). In so doing, the nurse manager must identify aspects of the organization's philosophy, goals, and objectives that may help or hinder the type of performance appraisal plan being evolved.

Thus, use of the inventory checklist becomes a minimanagement audit, investigating in a significant way the beliefs, attitudes, and values of the organization's administrators and managers as translated into operating techniques.

Clearly, past and present management practices throughout the organization influence the success of the performance appraisal program in nursing. Similarly, successful management innovations in the nursing department can have a beneficial influence on all other hospital departments. The inventory checklist therefore should be used carefully but thoroughly. The experience of completing the inventory will help the task force members to "think organizationally"—a most useful conceptual skill for nurse managers and practitioners. However, the team should not strive for too much detail or perfection in carrying out the process. It is important to get the job done with dispatch.

To paraphrase a well-known saying, "If a thing is worth doing it is worth doing. . . . poorly." Of course it is worth doing things well, but if striving for a concept of perfection or excellence is likely to delay implementation efforts unduly, then it is advisable to settle for a more rapidly obtainable standard of "satisfactory" or "OK."

So it is not necessary to make a big production of the nursing organization inventory checklist. The manager should wade into it, wade through it, get it done. Items that require more attention or development should be identified and assigned for follow-through. Then the manager and team can move ahead with the challenging work of shaping up the performance appraisal program itself.

RECOGNIZING AND DEALING WITH A DILEMMA

At this point, Albert Low's challenging writing on creative management is a valid resource. His wide research and executive experience provide new perspectives on management and organizational problems. For example, he introduces the subject of understanding and resolving a managerial dilemma with a discussion of the nature of work. He contrasts the physical energy expended in physical work with mental work—thinking. As he points out, "Thinking things through is hard work, coming to a decision is hard work, even thinking about work is hard." He asks why this is so and comes to some conclusions that can be of value to nurse managers in their roles with performance appraisal programs (Low, 1976):

> *To do mental work it is necessary to face and resolve a dilemma,* and it is because of this that work is hard. If there were no dilemma, there would be no mental work, but because there is a dilemma, work is necessary. . . . a recognizable pattern underlies work. This pattern is the pattern of a dilemma. (p. 141) [Emphasis in original]

Low describes the forces at work in a dilemma as those that on one hand repel each other but in other combinations attract each other. Comprehending these forces means understanding the two tendencies at work within a holon. He describes a holon as Janus-faced, having two faces, one inward and the other outward, each with two horns, with the characteristics of being both a part and a whole. The first two horns of the dilemma are concerned with internal, integrative aspects of the holon. The second two horns involve its external, assertive aspects. A system can be viewed from the point of view of structure as well as process, as in Figure 3-2.

Low offers an example of an administrative system dilemma that involves a salary administrator who is asked to set up a salary administration system (and thus it is highly pertinent to this book). The forces at work in this dilemma are as indicated in Figure 3-3. Low explains:

> When a salary administrator sets up a system he has to recognize that it is but one of a number of systems that the company needs. He must therefore devise a system that will cost as little as possible in terms of resources and management time for setting it up and for operating it. The more streamlined it is, the better.

> On the other hand, the salary administration system must be as complete as possible; all relevant jobs must be included. For example, if the system is designed for clerical employees, it is unwise to leave out some clerical jobs simply because of the difficulty of including them in the study. Furthermore, all relevant facts must be collected about all the jobs that are involved, and

Figure 3-2 Forces at Work in a Dilemma

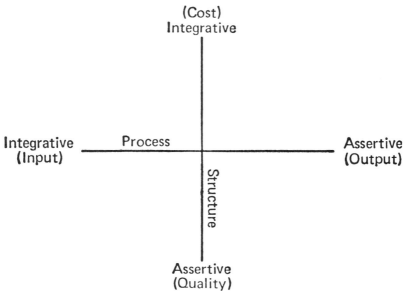

Figure 3-3 Administrative System Dilemma

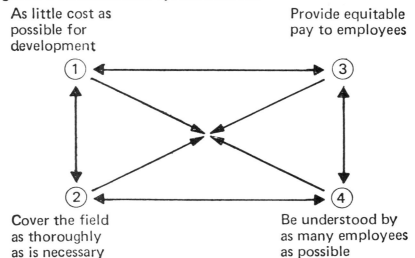

again it would be unwise to deliberately omit relevant facts because of the difficulty or cost of collecting them.

There is, therefore, an antagonism between these two considerations. . . . The more complete the system, the higher the cost is likely to be. The simpler the system, the more likely it is that something will be left out.

In addition, the system must be designed so that it gives satisfaction to those whose salaries are governed by it. One of the requirements of these people is that the salaries are administered equitably, the other is that they understand the system; that is, equity is perceived as such. However, these two requirements are in conflict.

Equity is obtained by ensuring that different levels of work are rewarded by correspondingly different levels of pay. Complete equity would prevail when each role had found its exact position in a pay hierarchy. Ideally, this would require a different level of pay for each role. But to explain to an employee why his salary is paid at one level and a colleague's at a slightly different level when the difference between the two roles is barely perceptible is a difficult problem. This problem of explanation is also highlighted when it is remembered that there is always a borderline case whenever one tries to divide a continuum into segments.

Equality is easier to talk about than equity—people understand equality better than equity. Unions have a tendency to want to erode pay differentials as it is easier to communicate equality to the rank and file. The same reason explains why dollars and cents rather than percentage increases are discussed. Dollar and cent increases tend toward equality; percentage increases tend toward equity. Equity, therefore, tends toward one grade for each job, while equality tends toward one grade for all jobs. Again this is a conflict.

Thus, in the illustration of this system [Figure 3-3], corners 1 and 2 are in opposition and so are corners 3 and 4. Corners 1 and 4, however, are complementary. The less complex the system, the easier it is to communicate. In fact, people often say, "Let's keep it simple," meaning "Let's make it easy to communicate." Corners 2 and 3 are complementary. The more complete and thorough, the greater the chance of equity being reached.

Furthermore, there are two internal aspects concerned with the system and two external aspects concerned with acceptance of the system: the first two concern the make-up of the system, the second two, the reception that others give it. (pp. 146–148) [A full set of salary administration dilemmas is given in Appendix 3-A at the end of this chapter.]

A worthwhile exercise is to review the salary administration dilemmas summarized in that Appendix. It includes the dilemmas of the total system, of job description, of job evaluation, and of writing the policy. The dilemmas of setting up performance appraisal and merit rating plans are not included. Thus, a pertinent exercise for the performance appraisal task force or committee is to think through the dilemmas of performance appraisal using the same models as those shown. The following additional material will be helpful in doing this exercise.

THE BASIC DILEMMA

Low demonstrates the value of having a general paradigm that would be useful as a means of identifying the specific dilemma underlying any particular work:

> This would make the dilemma conscious. At present a manager must deal with a dilemma at an unconscious, and therefore inarticulate, level. The solutions he comes to may be correct, but because they are inarticulate they cannot be adequately communicated, nor, often, are they as simple as they could be if they were exposed to the light of conscious reason. (p. 148).

> . . . A theory, organization, or system could be judged by reference to four criteria: simplicity, completeness, pragmatism, and communicability. These can be related to our paradigm as in Figure 3-4. Let us consider an organization to be a system that must be simple, complete, pragmatic, and communicable, and then let us see how it improves our understanding of the problem of organization and the nature of the dilemma.

> Organization is simple when there is no overlap between positions and therefore no redundancy in the system. Organization is complete when all work that should be done is done. The more complete the organization, the more complex it is likely to be. The more complexity, the greater the chance of territorial conflict. The simpler the organization, the less chance of conflict, but the greater the chances of something being left undone.

Figure 3-4 The 4 Criteria of Organization

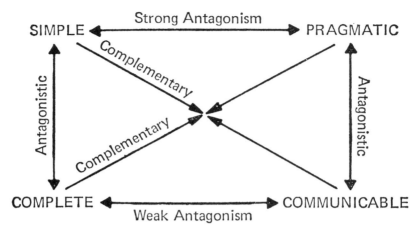

Source: Reprinted from Zen and Creative Management by Albert Low with permision of Doubleday & Company, Inc., © 1976 by Albert Low, p. 149.

What we have said can be illustrated by the product-function opposition, which is a common problem encountered in organization. A basic problem that arises in organization is whether delegation of work should be made in terms of the "product" [read, service] or the "function." "The dilemma of product versus function is by no means new; managers have been facing the same basic question for decades" (Walker & Lorsche, 1968, p. 130). "Corporations, especially manufacturers, have long wrestled with the problem of how to structure their organizations to enable employees, particularly specialists, to do their jobs with maximum efficiency and productivity. One perplexing issue has been whether to organize around functions or products." (Ibid, p. 129)

The question is whether specialists "in a given function, should be grouped under a common boss, regardless of the differences in products they are involved in, or should the various functional specialists, working on a single product, be grouped together under the same superior." (Ibid, p. 130) (Low, 1976, pp. 150–151)

It takes no stretch of the imagination to relate this to the organizational concerns of nurse administrators and hospital chief executive officers. Low concludes:

Corners 1 and 2 of the dilemma paradigm (Figure 3-4) represent the integrative mode of the holon viewed along the process dimension. (See also Figure 3-2.) Thus, simplicity and completeness concern the way that roles, tasks, operations, and functions are delegated. They are concerned with the *efficiency* of the system. Corners 3 and 4, representing the pragmatic and communication aspects, form the assertive mode and concern the output of these roles, the self-transcendent aspect of the holon, and the *effectiveness* of the system. (p. 151)

THE CIRCLE COMPLETED

This brief review of some of Albert Low's contributions brings the subject around full circle. (See Chapter 1, 15 Criteria for performance appraisal.) There is more to Low's comments than meets the eye upon first reading. They are included here because of their significance to the subject of organizing for performance appraisal. They serve also as a reminder that performance appraisal is only one management technique in a wage and salary administration program that exists within the complex management system of the total hospital organization.

Performance appraisal always has posed dilemmas. It has not always received the mental work to face and resolve it as a dilemma. It is to be hoped that nurse managers will continue to prepare themselves for the hard thinking required to resolve in their own situations the dilemma of performance appraisal.

For Discussion Purposes

Some members of your performance appraisal task force now wonder whether they should have agreed to serve. There is general agreement that performance appraisal is a more complex subject with broader implications than first realized. But everyone agrees to carry out the nursing department organization inventory using the checklist provided. In addition, there is some sentiment in favor of using Low's models for clarifying the dilemma of performance appraisal.

Describe how you would proceed with these additional steps, who would be invited to participate, and what target dates you would set for completion.

NOTES

Deines, E. *Staffing for DRGs: A unit-specific approach for nursing managers*. Chapel Hill, N.C.: W.L. Ganong Co., 1983.

Ganong, J.M., & Ganong, W.L. *HELP for the head nurse* (4th ed.). Chapel Hill, N.C.: W.L. Ganong Co., 1981.

Ganong, J.M., & Ganong, W.L. *HELP with career ladders in nursing*. Chapel Hill, N.C.: W.L. Ganong Co., 1982.

Ganong, J.M., & Ganong, W.L. The G-Gram Newsletter for Nurse Managers and Educators. Chapel Hill, N.C.: W.L. Ganong Co., March–April 1983, *10*(2), 3.

Lewin, K. *Field theory in social science*. Dorwin Cartwright (Ed.). New York: Harper and Brothers, 1951.

Low, A. *Zen and creative management*. Garden City, N.Y.: Anchor Press/Doubleday, 1976.

Meissner, W. "Theories of personality." in A.M. Nicholi (Ed.). *The Harvard Guide to Modern Psychiatry*, Cambridge, Mass.: The Belknap Press of Harvard University, 1978, p. 136.

Toffler, A. *Future shock*. New York: Bantam Books, Inc., 1974.

Walker, A.H., & Lorsche, J.W. Organizational choice: Product vs. function. *Harvard Business Review*, November–December 1968, *46*(6), 129–138.

Appendix 3-A

Dilemmas Involved in Setting Up a Salary Administration System

TOTAL SYSTEM

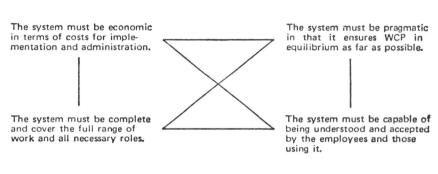

The system must be economic in terms of costs for implementation and administration.

The system must be pragmatic in that it ensures WCP in equilibrium as far as possible.

The system must be complete and cover the full range of work and all necessary roles.

The system must be capable of being understood and accepted by the employees and those using it.

In practice this dilemma is expressed as:

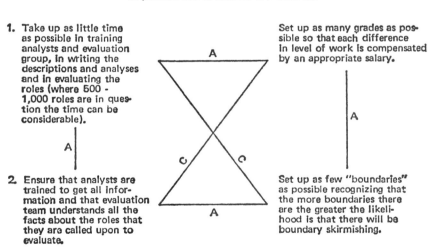

1. Take up as little time as possible in training analysts and evaluation group, in writing the descriptions and analyses and in evaluating the roles (where 500 - 1,000 roles are in question the time can be considerable).

Set up as many grades as possible so that each difference in level of work is compensated by an appropriate salary.

2. Ensure that analysts are trained to get all information and that evaluation team understands all the facts about the roles that they are called upon to evaluate.

Set up as few "boundaries" as possible recognizing that the more boundaries there are the greater the likelihood is that there will be boundary skirmishing.

Appendix 3-A continued

DILEMMAS OF JOB DESCRIPTION

1. Job Description should be as simple as possible each statement being succinct and independent of other statements. (It should follow a basic convention in order that differences in description format alone should not imply a difference in content or level, descriptions should involve as little work as possible.)

2. Job description and analysis must contain as much detail as necessary in order to capture the spirit as well as the content of the role as well as to satisfy the incumbent that sufficient is known of his role to enable an adequate evaluation to be made.

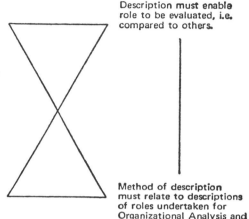

Description must enable role to be evaluated, i.e. compared to others.

Method of description must relate to descriptions of roles undertaken for Organizational Analysis and Role Specifications.

DILEMMAS OF JOB EVALUATION

Use as straightforward and simple an evaluation system and factors as possible to cut down costs in training, explaining and administering.

Use as sophisticated an evaluation procedure as necessary in order to take into account role differences.

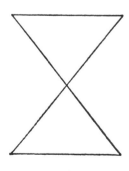

Involve as few people in the evaluation process as possible in order to simplify the program. If there are too many involved, it becomes difficult to schedule meetings and to maintain a consistency of judgment as well as there being a greater likelihood of group pressure building up.

Involve as many people in the evaluation process as necessary in order to gain acceptance of the system. Each group in the company should feel that it is represented in the group.

Appendix 3-A continued

DILEMMAS IN WRITING THE POLICY

Set up as simple a policy as possible with as few exceptions and special considerations as possible. Alter as infrequently as possible, each alteration calling for more training, further adjustment and increased likelihood for misunderstanding.

Ensure policy takes into account local problems and local differences. Establish differential grade where possible.

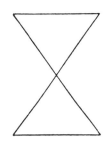

Put in as much detail as necessary and word as tightly as necessary to avoid ambiguity and points being overlooked. Loose wording leads to a steady erosion of policy and allows "gray" areas to develop.

Ensure that policy is as "human" as possible to allow people to understand it. One of the most frequent criticisms of Salary Administration Systems is that they are too esoteric.

Source: Reprinted from *Zen and Creative Management* by Albert Low with permission of Doubleday & Company, Inc., © by Albert Low, Appendix II.

Chapter 4

A Productivity-Oriented Performance Appraisal Program

INTRODUCTION TO ROPEP

Nurse managers today generally recognize their key role in productivity. They know, too, that there rarely seems to be enough time to manage as well as they know how. Thus they do not welcome complicated, time-consuming performance appraisal techniques. They need an easy-to-use method that helps them and their people focus on optimal performance results consistent with unit and organizational goals.

This chapter presents such a method. It can be adapted to the specific purposes that performance appraisal is intended to serve in each organization. In addition, it is designed to facilitate the initiation of career ladders (as described in Chapter 6). In fact, the most economical and effective approach is to develop job performance descriptions that include the type of standards and levels-of-performance criteria that serve the mutual needs of appraisal and career ladders. Examples of a number of such applications are included in the appendixes.

ROPEP is the acronym for a Results-Oriented Performance Evaluation Program. The term performance evaluation as used in connection with ROPEP and productivity is defined as *the measurement of the results of a person's work effort compared with previously agreed-upon standards of performance*. This definition is broad enough to apply to the employee performance appraisal process at all job levels in every type of organization. It is specific enough to differentiate it from the variety of other terms used as synonyms.

More specifically, *performance evaluation* (appraisal) is the *measurement* (the determination of the degree of conformity with criteria of quality and quantity) of the *results* (consequences, outcomes) of a person's *work effort* (on-the-job activities and exertion) *compared* (examined in order to note the similarities or differences) with previously *agreed-upon* (jointly developed in advance with accord by the manager and the employee) *standards* (acknowledged measures of comparison for qualitative or quantitative value; criteria; norms).

The introduction of an important performance evaluation program such as ROPEP in the nursing department or division is sometimes long delayed, awaiting a top-level administrative exploration, decision, and hospitalwide implementation effort. This is unfortunate because more often than not there is no need for a uniform plan in all departments. In fact, there may be valid reasons for using varied approaches, different starting dates, and different implementation steps in different departments.

Guidelines and specific implementation steps for ROPEP that can be used by nurse managers involve four phases:

Phase I   Initial Development
Phase II   Introduction
Phase III   First Evaluation Cycle
Phase IV   Continuing Evaluation Cycle

These are presented in sequence, the first two in this chapter, Phases III and IV in Chapter 5.

INITIAL DEVELOPMENT, PHASE I

The development of a results-oriented performance evaluation program usually begins with selecting a working group (a committee, task force, or project team) that is charged with responsibility for the system's overall design. One of its early activities is to prepare the program performance plan and work sheet. Figure 4-1 is an example of such a form.

Performance, Not Job, Descriptions

ROPEP requires the preparation of performance descriptions rather than the conventional job descriptions. Sometimes called job performance descriptions, these look different from the usual performance descriptions because they are different. They are organized differently because their focus is on performance responsibilities of specific persons and on standards of performance for each key performance responsibility. They were designed this way originally (in the late 1960s) because the authors recognized the need for a sound management approach to making each person on the nursing staff accountable for the quality of patient care.

Job descriptions and performance descriptions are basically different because they are developed for two different purposes. The job descrip-

Figure 4-1 ROPEP: Program Performance Plan and Work Sheet

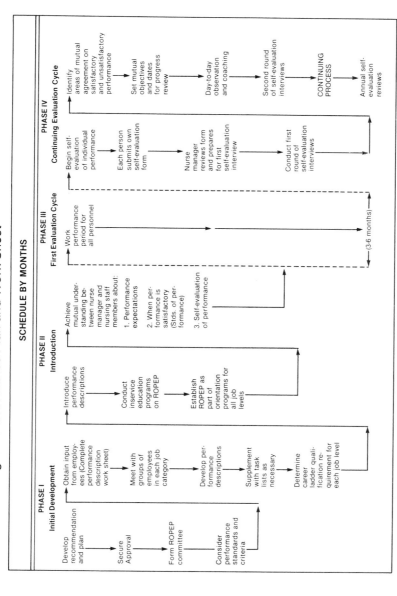

Source: Reprinted from *HELP with Performance Appraisal: A Results-Oriented Approach* by Joan M. Ganong and Warren L. Ganong with permission of W.L. Ganong Co., 1981, p. 105.

tion, by its very title, describes a job. It is prepared by a process of job analysis. Its purpose is primarily to provide the descriptive job information necessary for evaluation—establishing the relative worth (pay) of jobs. A performance description, by contrast, describes performance responsibilities and standards. As noted in Chapter 3, it is prepared by a process of performance analysis carried out by employees with their own managers (supervisors, department heads, bosses). Its purpose is to reach agreement and understanding between employees and their managers regarding the former's performance responsibilities and specific performance criteria so that meaningful, continuing evaluation can take place, leading to optimal quality/quantity effectiveness and productivity.

A performance description by definition is a statement of the purpose of a person's function within the organization, the major performance responsibilities (grouped by persons to whom the responsibilities exist), and measures of satisfactory performance. The emphasis in preparation is on reaching mutual understandings between employees and managers regarding who is to do what for whom, when, and how well so that there can be later understanding and agreement regarding what was done for whom, when, and how well.

This is the sine qua non of achieving individual accountability for optimal quality and productivity. The appendix includes examples of performance descriptions as well as job descriptions that have been modified to include criteria-based performance standards.

Completion of a performance description work sheet is an important way to help personnel understand the performance requirements (Exhibit 4-1). This type of work sheet, to be completed by every employee in every job, provides for valuable input by the people who know the most about their performance responsibilities—namely, those who are doing the work. When all of the responses from all of the employees with the same job title are summarized, a wealth of information is available for preparing a meaningful first draft of the major performance responsibilities for that particular job—as described by the employees themselves. Similarly, employees' answers to the question, "How do you know when you are doing a good job?" provide excellent clues to their perceptions of satisfactory performance.

The Process Begins

The performance description work sheets can be distributed by nurse managers at small departmental or unit meetings. Their purpose can be explained, with time for questions and answers. It is helpful to state their

Exhibit 4-1 Performance Description Work Sheet

NAME: _____ DEPT: _____

JOB TITLE: _____ DATE: _____

Name of your supervisor: _____

Name of your department head: _____

Names and titles of persons you supervise (if you are a supervisor or manager):

_____   _____

_____   _____

_____   _____

_____   _____

    INSTRUCTIONS: You can help prepare an up-to-date Performance Description of what you do in your work. Please be as complete as possible. Do not be bashful; list everything you think is part of your job. If you need more space, use additional sheets.

1. The purpose of my work is _____

_____

_____

2. For whom are you doing your work? _____

_____

_____

3. How do you know whether or not you are performing your work satisfactorily? _____

_____

4. List anything you are doing that you think *should not* be part of your work: _____

_____

5. List anything you are *not* doing that you think *should* be part of your work: _____

_____

6. Who taught you your work? _____

7. When you started your present job, how long did it take you to learn to do the work satisfactorily? _____

8. COMMENTS & SUGGESTIONS: Add anything else that will help your work and how you feel about it. (Use additional sheets if you need more space): _____

_____

_____

_____

_____

_____

LIST THE MAIN THINGS YOU DO AS PART OF YOUR DAILY WORK

_____   _____

_____   _____

Exhibit 4-1 continued

(Use additional sheets if you need more space)

LIST OTHER THINGS YOU DO BUT THAT DO NOT HAPPEN EVERY DAY

Source: Reprinted from *HELP with Performance Appraisal: A Results-Oriented Approach* by Joan M. Ganong and Warren L. Ganong with permission of W.L. Ganong Co.,© 1981, pp. 25–26.

purpose directly on the work sheet forms, with instructions for completing them. This will minimize misunderstandings.

Upon completion, these work sheets should be signed in order to strengthen the most important of all on-the-job relationships—that of trust between employees and managers. Anonymous questionnaires smack too much of the kind of gameplaying that ROPEP seeks to eliminate. Admittedly there may be some organizational circumstances that might indicate unsigned responses when the work sheets are used for the first time. Whenever this is the case, it is symptomatic of significant administrative, supervisory, or labor relations problems that deserve attention before ROPEP is introduced. As a matter of fact, a potent remedial action for such problems is a well-planned implementation of the entire ROPEP process, beginning at the top administrative level.

Once the job performance work sheets have been accumulated they should be sorted by job title and the responses summarized and analyzed.

Information from the forms includes significant perceptions and opinions about specific responsibilities and activities. As the analysis continues, patterns will emerge that can be helpful in formulating the first draft of a job performance description for each job title.

Before any attempt is made to write a draft, however, the summaries should be discussed with small groups of employees to amplify and clarify some of the information. This is another opportunity for the nurse manager and employees to continue trust building through open discussion. It is important to look for items of general agreement rather than exceptions to the group consensus.

Information from the work sheets also can be helpful in developing or expanding a skills list. This is a comprehensive listing of procedures, techniques, and skills required as individuals carry out their responsibilities. To avoid cluttering the job performance description, these skills lists can be a separate addendum.

A job performance description may go through several drafts before it is finally agreed to by employees, the committee, and nursing administration. The final draft should include the position title; the division or department name; the titles of the employees supervised; the person to whom the individual reports; the date it is initiated, reviewed, and/or revised; a brief statement of the purpose of the job or its primary function; the performance responsibilities; and the behavioral criteria for standards of satisfactory performance. To be complete, it also should list qualifications, identified as those that are *required* of anyone aspiring to the job as well as those that are *desirable*.

Formats: No One Best Style

Experience teaches that there is no one best format for these descriptions. A two-column format (Exhibit 4-2) is suggested for simplicity, ease of reading, and understanding. Another format is an outline style, with the criteria indented under each responsibility, which in turn may be organized under the person to whom the responsibility exists. Examples of several formats can be found in the appendix.

The actual writing of the first draft of a job performance description should be done by a single individual who has writing skills. It is wasteful of time and effort to attempt such drafts by committee. Once the draft has been written, it can be critiqued by committee members as well as by representatives of the people whose lives it will affect most (the specific employee groups). Then successive drafts can be written that include acceptable changes.

Exhibit 4-2 Two-Column Job Performance Format

Major Performance Responsibilities	Performance Standards & Criteria
	Performance is satisfactory when:
To Patients (or other agency clients)	(For each item, a statement is made of the measurable conditions that
To Medical Staff	will exist when performance is sat-
To Own Nurse Manager	isfactory.)
To Unit Personnel	
To Committees	
To Other Department Personnel	
To Other Organizations	
To Self	

Source: Reprinted from *HELP with Performance Appraisal: A Results-Oriented Approach* by Joan M. Ganong and Warren L. Ganong with permission of W.L. Ganong Co., © 1981, p. 20.

The two-column format of Exhibit 4-2 can be helpful in identifying the persons *to whom* the individual job holder has responsibilities, naming the key responsibilities, and describing the criteria for satisfactory performance. The major responsibilities should be written concisely and should indicate clearly what is expected of the individual. The right-hand column lists, for each performance responsibility, the specific behaviors (or results, outcomes) that serve as criteria against which to measure whether or not the performance of that responsibility is satisfactory.

Criteria are defined as standards on which a judgment can be based. Obviously, they are used as a means of judging. They serve as an acknowledged measure of comparison for both quantitative and qualitative values. These *criteria* can best be described, when they appear in a job performance description, as identified behaviors that are observable when they are being performed or when the documented results of them are observable in a patient's medical record.

Broadly speaking, standards of performance are written statements that define, and provide a measure of, how well employees are expected to carry out their responsibilities and meet their objectives. Some confusion with terminology is caused by the fact that standard and criterion are synonyms. They have been defined separately here so that standards refer to the broader, more goal-oriented descriptors and criterion to the highly objective, specific, behavioral descriptors. Examples of such job performance descriptions are included in the apendixes.

As a precautionary note, numbers-minded nurse managers will do well to heed the advice of Beaulieu (cited early in Chapter 2 in connection with *Assumption No. 4*). "The illusive pursuit of ways to measure the unmeasurable is avoided when it is recognized that the locus is *verification,* not quantification. Means of verifying accomplishments are far easier to arrive at than are rigidly quantifiable measurements. The performance standard that eludes verification has not yet presented itself."

Guidelines for Writing Measurable Behaviors

Specific written behaviors are used to indicate to individuals what they are expected to do. These behaviors indicate when the individual is carrying out the major performance responsibilities in a satisfactory manner.

Time frames help specify requirements such as "at least every two hours," "at least once a shift," "no more than once a week." Other numbers can be used also as part of the time frames. Examples might be: "Attends at least three assigned committee meetings per month;" or "Is late no more than once per month;" or "Completes and documents at least one evaluation of patient progress every eight hours."

Percentages are used to place minimums and maximums in perspective. Examples are: "A minimum of 75 percent of meetings are attended annually;" "Prepares and documents a beginning care plan for assigned patients at least 95 percent of time."

"Each" and "every" are used to quantify behavioral criteria. Examples include: "Completes assessment for each assigned patient," "Attends every meeting." The use of *procedures* and *techniques* simplifies the wording of the behavioral criteria: "Completes discharge summary form for every patient according to procedure;" or "Listens to breath sounds using correct technique."

Measurable statements using these examples and guidelines can be used singly or in combination. These statements are intended to assist both the manager and the employee to understand the expected behavior clearly. It is an attempt to avoid evaluating people on personality traits and focus instead on observable and measurable performance behaviors.

Results, Productivity, and Competence

The nurse manager has the right to expect from an appraisal program that it be results/productivity oriented. That is, that it will measure the results of a person's work effort as compared with previously agreed-upon standards and criteria and encourage changes in behavior that are necessary to make that performance satisfactory if it is not so already.

Much emphasis continues on seeking productive, effective behavior. Productivity in nursing means yielding favorable, useful results. As much importance is placed on outcomes as on outputs. Such outcomes should accrue to the patient and family but also to staff personnel.

Psychologists have defined a productive orientation as a healthy outlook that permits individuals to be creative in work as well as in social relations and to use well whatever potentialities they possess (English & English, 1958, p. 411). A productive orientation also has been referred to as an attitude or personal anticipation that the "prospects are good that competent performance will yield the psychological rewards associated with competence, feelings of efficacy and of self-worth" (Hall, 1980, p. 48).

In a health care setting it is imperative that the individual worker demonstrate competency, which by dictionary definition means to be "adequate for the purpose: suitable; sufficient" (American Heritage, 1973, p. 271). In that sense the individual nurse must be able to carry out competently the behaviors that are cited in the job performance description criteria. In addition to this view of competence, however, there has to be something in it for the individual nurse. Hall (1980, p. 35) refers to a competence motive as a need among people to demonstrate their competence and behave in a competent manner. This is done not just for the sake of the work itself but to meet the basic human need for self-worth. Nurse managers will do well to look upon the appraisal process as an opportunity to enhance and capitalize on such a motivational need.

In summary, a healthy work environment is one in which performance appraisals—based on specified responsibilities and behavioral criteria—foster in people a results orientation, a competency motivation, and productivity awareness. All of these are in the best interests of attaining the goals of the health care organization, the patients being served, and the personnel involved.

INTRODUCTION, PHASE II

Phase II of ROPEP begins with an introduction of the new job performance descriptions. With early involvement of the nursing staff and the nurse managers during the development phase, there should be no surprises when the new descriptions finally are completed and introduced. It is important that everyone understand that on an announced date the old job descriptions will be obsolete and the new job performance descriptions will be in effect.

Before that date, nurse managers must take three steps to:

1. conduct inservice education programs on ROPEP
2. establish ROPEP as a part of the orientation programs for all new employees
3. achieve mutual understanding between themselves and the nursing staff concerning the new job performance descriptions.

It is helpful to publicize the new performance appraisal program in newsletters, on bulletin boards, by word of mouth, and in memos. The public relations department or the person who handles such matters should be called upon during this phase to lend whatever assistance is necessary to promote the program.

Nurse managers at every level need to prepare to initiate the ROPEP program with their employees. This is a very important step. Its success rests heavily not just on what the nurse managers do but how they do it. Obviously, no two nurse managers will do this in the same way but it is important that each show enthusiasm and commitment for the program and explain the vital role of each employee.

Employees will be at different stages of readiness for such a program. Those who have had an opportunity to participate in preparing the work sheets and drafts of the job performance descriptions will be better prepared. However, newer employees, as well as those who for one reason or another did not participate in Phase I, will be less informed and may require more initial orientation.

In any event, emphasis must be placed on the self-evaluation feature of the program based on the major responsibilities and the performance criteria as stated in the job performance description. This is used with the evaluation by the nurse managers at the time evaluation conferences are held.

MANAGER'S GUIDE AND CHECKLIST

Exhibit 4-3 provides a nurse manager's guide and checklist for the use of job performance descriptions in role clarification and performance appraisal. An explanation of each item on the checklist follows. The manager should:

A. Meet with each employee to discuss and reach a mutual understanding of the employee's performance responsibilities and measures of satisfactory performance.

Exhibit 4-3 Manager's Guide and Checklist for the Use of Performance Descriptions in Role Clarification and in Performance Evaluation

---

An Employee Self-Evaluation Method

The manager will:

A. Meet with each employee to discuss and reach a mutual understanding of the employee's responsibilities and measures of satisfactory performance.

_____ 1. Review the performance description.
_____ 2. Ask for comments and questions.
_____ 3. Clarify and amplify the performance descriptions, through discussion.
_____ 4. Explain the self-evaluation procedure (including the exception principle).

B. Establish a plan for regular employee self-evaluation.

_____ 1. Set a date for completion of first self-evaluation.
_____ 2. Obtain from employees their own written comments regarding how well they think they are meeting each of their performance responsibilities. Exhibit 4-4 provides a useful form for this purpose.

C. Meet with employees individually to review their self-evaluations.

_____ 1. Set dates for the discussions.
_____ 2. Meet with the employees individually and listen to their comments.
_____ 3. Agree whenever possible with the employee's own evaluation of the major performance responsibilities.
_____ 4. When you disagree with the self-evaluation of a responsibility, ask the employees to explain again their reasons for their own evaluations. Then indicate why you feel that the performance results are better than, or not as good as, the employee's own evaluation.
_____ 5. Reach agreement upon those performance results that need strengthening.
_____ 6. Develop suggestions for improvement with the employee. Help identify available resources.
_____ 7. Agree upon specific follow-through action.

Source: Reprinted from *HELP with Performance Appraisal: A Results-Oriented Approach* by Joan M. Ganong and Warren L. Ganong with permission of W.L. Ganong Co., © 1981, p. 39.

---

1. Review the performance description.

This step is considerably simplified if the employee has helped to prepare the statements in the performance description. When that is the case, there may be a temptation to omit this first step on the assumption that it is not necessary. Such a temptation must be resisted. Circumstances change. Work experiences can change a person's viewpoints and interpretations. An individual's apperceptive mass continues to evolve. So while this first step may take less time with the employee who was involved in the first writing of the performance description, it always should be included with each individual as part of every periodic evaluation discussion.

2. Ask for comments and questions.

The intent in this step is to encourage an open, free-and-easy exploration of what the employee's work is all about—its purpose, what has to be done for whom, and so on. How managers bring about this kind of discussion depends greatly upon their own individual styles. What works well for one person may not work so well for another. A vital factor, however, that has a great influence on the level of communication that takes place is the attitude the managers bring to the discussion. This will be communicated and will influence what happens. Some tips for stimulating productive discussion are presented in the last section of this chapter, and in chapters 5 and 7.

3. Clarify and amplify the performance descriptions, through discussion.

This is especially essential for the first meeting with employees who have not previously seen the performance descriptions for their jobs. This cannot be hurried. Whatever time it takes will be well spent. (How long does it take and how much does it cost to process a grievance? A labor arbitration case? A lawsuit in court?)

The manager should ask repeatedly, "What does this mean to you?" "Tell me in your own words what this means." It also should be explained: "The reason we are doing this is so that both you and I have the same understanding about your work and what we can expect of each other." The manager should say, "What I think I heard you say was . . ." (repeat what employee said). "Do you mean that . . . ?" (try to give same message in different words of your own choosing). An example can illustrate the meaning: "For example, if a patient asks to be helped out of bed, then slips and falls on the floor, do you mean that you would . . . (etc)?"

4. Explain the self-evaluation procedure (including the exception principle).

The self-evaluation aspect of ROPEP is an element that requires emphasis throughout every step. The manager explains:

"The reason for our having this kind of a self-evaluation program is so that you can feel comfortable doing your work without having me looking over your shoulder. Most people don't like the idea of a manager being a 'snoopervisor.' I don't like it either. The best way for both of us to get along together is for us to understand what both of us (you and me) consider to be satisfactory performance of your responsibilities. So let's take a look at these again.''

The manager then should point out that the first regular evaluation discussion will include all of the performance responsibilities. Subsequent regular evaluations (once or twice a year) will focus on performance results that are exceptionally outstanding or exceptional because they do not meet the standard of satisfactory performance. This is the exception principle. All other performance results require no attention because they are satisfactory.

Performance evaluation really is a continuing day-to-day process. Thus, there are likely to be many occasions between regular evaluation review sessions when the performance descriptions will be used to clarify questions, remind each other of performance standards, help plan skill improvement programs, and for other work-related purposes.

B. Establish a plan for regular employee self-evaluation.

1. Set a date for completion of first self-evaluation.

This date may be set during the discussion in Step A-4. Much depends upon the readiness of the individual employees. One person may require more than one discussion to complete the first four steps, another may be ready to carry out the self-evaluation immediately following step A-4.

The manager will be able to judge how soon to allow the self-evaluation step to be completed, saying, for example, "How soon will you want to complete your first self-evaluation of performance?" There usually is no need to hurry it. For one person it may be within the month, for another, two or three months.

2. Obtain from employees their own written comments regarding how well they think they are meeting each of their performance responsibilities.

The manager must remind employees to include every performance responsibility in this first self-evaluation. They can use an extra copy of the performance description to record their comments. For subsequent evaluations, the form in Exhibit 4-4 may be used. Whatever form is used, the employee is expected to submit it to the manager by the date agreed upon.

Employees should be encouraged to discuss their efforts at self-evaluation with the manager if they wish to do so. They may need nothing more

Exhibit 4-4 Sample Self-Evaluation of Performance Results Form

SELF-EVALUATION OF PERFORMANCE RESULTS		
NAME: _____ DATE: _____		
TITLE: _____		
DEPARTMENT: _____ REPORTS TO: _____		

Instructions: First review your job performance description, especially the performance standards and criteria. Mark the items for which you think your results have been consistently satisfactory or unsatisfactory. Then check (✔) below your overall evaluation of results for A thru G as satisfactory (OK) or unsatisfactory (Not OK). Write your comments in the space provided; use additional sheets as needed.

PERFORMANCE RESULTS

	OK	NOT OK
A. To Patients		
B. To Medical Staff		
C. To Your Own Manager (supervisor)		
D. To Department Personnel		
E. To Committees		
F. To Personnel of Other Departments (or organizations)		
G. To Self		

Source: Reprinted from *HELP with Performance Appraisal: A Results-Oriented Approach* by Joan M. Ganong and Warren L. Ganong with permission of W.L. Ganong Co., © 1981, p. 20.

than to have some time to explain how they are progressing and to have support as to the kinds of words they are using. This can be highly valuable in preparing both employee and manager for a productive follow through.

C. Meet with employees individually to review their self-evaluations.

1. Set dates for the discussions.

Establishing and maintaining a schedule for evaluation discussions is an indication of the importance management attaches to this activity. Flexibility should be allowed in the time planned for each discussion so there will be no need to cut short a talk that is proving to be long but productive. Managers should schedule no more than one evaluation session on any one day.

2. Meet with employees individually and listen to their comments.

Even when the manager has the employee's written self-evaluation comments in advance of the discussion, there is merit in permitting the person to explain the analysis verbally. It is part of the process of maintaining a maximum level of communications and understanding at a most crucial point in the procedure.

3. Agree whenever possible with the employee's own evaluation of the major performance responsibilities.

The purpose of this procedure is to reach a meeting of the minds (the manager's and the employee's) regarding the latter's performance results. The manager should seek areas of agreement, not disagreement. The main question to be agreed upon for each responsibility is "Has performance been satisfactory or not satisfactory as measured against the stated criteria in the performance description?"

4. When you disagree with the self-evaluation of a responsibility, ask the employees to explain again their reasons for their own evaluations. Then indicate why you feel that the performance results are better than, or not as good as, the employee's own evaluation.

If both the employee and the manager have the same understanding of the responsibilities being evaluated and of the measures of satisfactory performance, then any disagreement would stem from differing knowledge of actual performance results (or differing interpretations of them). The process of examining each of these aspects in turn for any performance responsibility on which there appears to be a lack of agreement will minimize the likelihood of unnecessary misunderstandings.

The manager should maintain adequate personnel records to provide backup factual data for any unsatisfactory performance as well as for an exceptionally good one. Such documentation is essential for a number of valid purposes related to accreditation standards, nursing audit, patient care, lawsuits, labor relations when unions are involved, and effective personnel administration. One of the useful documentation methods is the critical incident technique. This is a factual approach for gathering information based on direct observation. An incident is any observable bit of human behavior sufficiently complete in itself to permit inferences to be made about the person performing the act (Fivars and Gosnell, 1966, p. 16).

5. *Reach agreement upon those performance results that need strengthening.*

This step is not always necessary with all employees for every regular performance evaluation. One of the fallacies in evaluation practices is the idea that there always is something wrong with employees or with their performance. Rating forms frequently seem to encourage emphasis on weaknesses rather than strengths. It thus is no wonder the appraisal procedure has such a bad reputation.

It is not necessary to make a special effort to find evidence of poor performance results that require improvement. Managers need not feel that they are poor evaluators if they cannot always identify weaknesses in employees' performances. On the contrary, they should take credit when they have provided the kind of training and leadership that minimizes or eliminates below-satisfactory results.

However, when outcomes have been less than satisfactory, they must be faced for what they are. It is to be hoped that both manager and employee will recognize and agree upon the evidence of unsatisfactory work. Whenever there is a lack of such agreement, and the manager is convinced that the results for a given major performance responsibility clearly are unsatisfactory, then that evaluation must be made known to the employee. The manager then must proceed in whatever manner is most likely to assure the desired level of performance.

6. *Develop suggestions for improvement with the employee. Help identify available resources.*

As with the preceding item, this is not always a necessary part of the self-evaluation process with all employees. Significant numbers of them are likely to be delivering satisfactory performance for all of their major responsibilities. Many are valuable in their present jobs, have no need to improve, and have no desire to qualify for higher paid positions. They form an important and usually stable portion of the work force. They are using their assets well and deserve credit for doing so.

When improvement is required on one or more performance responsibilities, the employee is asked, "What do you want to do about it?" Whatever improvement is to occur has to come about through the efforts of the individuals. They have to motivate themselves to make improved performance happen. The manager can suggest sources of help and guidance when it is wanted and, when necessary, can prescribe the needed remedy.

7. Agree upon specific follow-through action.

This is the specific outcome of a regular performance self-evaluation discussion. This step answers the questions, "What happens now? What do we do next?"

For some employees the follow-through is signified by the manager's parting comment, "Keep up the good work." For others there will be an understanding of agreed-upon action by the employees (and perhaps the manager also) that will lead to the correction of the unsatisfactory performance. This agreement should be in writing and should follow the general pattern of the management by objectives technique—set a goal, set a date, evaluate. Exhibit 5-1 in Chapter 5 provides a simple way to record this information for future follow-through.

APPRAISAL INTERVIEWING GUIDELINES

Interviewing is a communication process. Communication is the creation of understanding. A variety of skills are involved. How they are used depends upon the purpose, perception, and ability of the interviewer.

Observing an employee means to pay attention through the use of the key senses of sight, hearing, and touch. Observing also means being alert to the feeling tones perceivable from a person. Observing is a part of the communication process. Following are guidelines for interviewing.

A. General Guidelines

1. The climate the manager sets influences the interview. The manager should:

- Welcome the employee by name and clarify the reason for the interview.
- Make sure both parties are seated comfortably during the session.
- Show a sincere interest in what the employee is saying; listen attentively.
- Establish trust by proximity, responsiveness, openness, attention, privacy, confidentiality, honesty.
- Determine the employee's feelings and knowledge as effectively, efficiently, and pleasantly as possible.
- Present an attitude of warm acceptance and understanding coupled with objectivity; this enhances the results of an interview.

The manager also should:

2. Always use the job performance responsibilities and criteria as the basis for the interview; do not rely on memory; use notes; have specific information.
3. Remember that the needs and goals of both employee and nurse manager determine the purpose and outcome of an interview.
4. Do not ask questions of the employee that are answered elsewhere already unless it is necessary to check for accuracy.
5. Keep the interview on the track.
6. Follow the structure of an appraisal interview: the welcome, moving through and keeping on track, agreeing on goals and objectives, and bringing closure. (See Table 5-1 in Chapter 5.)
7. Focus on the employee's behavior rather than on the person; a manager who does not like the person's "attitude" should give specific instances of behavior rather than focussing on "attitude."
8. Practice interviewing to refine use of the technique and help identify and correct weak spots in such skills; the more interviews are conducted, the more adept the manager can become.

B. Use of Questions

The manager should:

1. Use direct questions to get specific information:

   - "What is your objective target date?"
   - "When did you complete that inservice program?"

2. Use exploratory questions to encourage further comments and expression of feeling:

- "How do you feel about that?"
- "Would you tell me more about that?"

3. Use open-ended questions to allow comment on whatever is on the employee's mind:

- "What would you like to talk about?"
- "How can I help you to change that behavior?"

C. Listening

The manager should:

1. Listen for facts and for meanings.
2. Concentrate on the employee and what the individual is saying.
3. Don't be afraid of silence; wait long enough for a response in the employee's own way.
4. Listen, then write; take time for eye contact.
5. Listen responsively and thoughtfully.
6. Remember: *Meanings are in people, not in words.*

D. Use of Specific Information

The manager can say:

1. "An audit of your assigned patients' charts shows only 10 out of 20 to have updated nursing care plans for the first two weeks of this month. This is an unacceptable pattern of behavior."
2. "You have attended and participated in every patient care conference over the past three months. This is a fine example of meeting and exceeding the criterion."

E. Use of the Senses

The manager should:

1. Look for reaction to conversation, eye contact, responsiveness, open use of specific information.

2. Watch facial expressions to pick up clues about such things as pleasure, fear, doubt, anxiety, satisfaction, anger, hostility, and confidence.
3. Watch body posture and position for clues about the points just mentioned.
4. Clarify any assumptions made from what is observed.
5. Listen for the timbre of a person's voice, the emphasis placed on words, for unspoken questions and needs.

F. Additional Guidelines for Observing

The manager should:

1. Remember that it is easy to *see* without *observing,* so attention must be paid to detail.
2. Observe for willingness to concentrate on specific predetermined criteria.
3. Observe by looking at the employee holistically.
4. Take time to be receptive to what the senses are saying; observe receptively.
5. Remember, in observing the employee, that what is observed depends on the manager; "What you *see* may be what you *expect to see.*"
6. Remember that people's behavior stems from their interpretation of what they think they perceive.
7. Practice observing silently to allow all of the receptive senses to function without interfering vocally.
8. Observe for information; observing includes reading.

G. Other Communication Skills

The manager should use the sum total of all verbal and nonverbal communication skills during an interview. People use the movements of their head, arms, eyes, and torso to punctuate their speech and to communicate additional meanings.

For Discussion Purposes

Members of your performance appraisal task force now are taking the bit in their teeth. They realize that what they have been engaged in would be part of Phase I of an orderly plan for introducing a results-oriented, criteria-based performance evaluation plan. They realize also that the existing performance appraisal plan may contain some components worth keeping.

Some members are insistent that they want the performance appraisal process itself to be as simple as possible. They may want major emphasis to be placed on the careful development of job performance descriptions that will clarify role requirements and facilitate an in-house (or system-wide) career ladder program with criteria-based, behaviorally oriented levels-of-performance definitions for each step on each ladder. This poses additional dilemmas.

1. Describe these dilemmas.
2. Suggest how to resolve them.
3. Recommend how to utilize the program performance plan and work sheet (Figure 4-1, supra) to facilitate the process.

NOTES

American Heritage Dictionary of the English Language. New York: American Heritage Publishing Co., 1973.

English, H., & English, A. *A comprehensive dictionary of psychological and psychoanalytical terms.* New York: Longmans, Green, Inc., 1958.

Fivars, G., & Gosnell, D. *Nursing evaluation: The problem and the process.* New York: Macmillan Publishing Co., Inc., 1966.

Ganong, J.M., & Ganong, W.L. *HELP with performance appraisal: A results-oriented approach.* Chapel Hill, N.C.: W.L. Ganong Co., 1981.

Hall, J. *The competence process: Managing for commitment and creativity.* The Woodlands, Texas: Teleometrics, 1980.

Chapter 5

Using the ROPEP System

THE FIRST EVALUATION CYCLE, PHASE III

Phase III, the first evaluation cycle, follows the introductory stage of the Results-Oriented Performance Evaluation Program (ROPEP). It is the time during which the employees begin working under the new job performance descriptions. It also is a time when nurse managers will do well to keep reiterating the newly defined responsibilities and criteria as the transition proceeds. Time has to be allowed for this transition. Success depends on how involved the employees have been in the design of the program.

Prior discussion has emphasized that job performance descriptions are the final outcome of the combined efforts of nurse managers and employees. Reaching mutual understanding and agreement on job performance responsibilities and criteria is as important as the actual wording of the statements that are used in the final form of the job performance description itself.

Once such understanding is achieved, the interpretation of the words and the meanings of the descriptions are likely to be more uniform. When such mutual understanding is lacking, agreement on the other phases of the program becomes much more difficult. Phase III, when the new job performance descriptions actually come into use, is the time when all the fruits of employee involvement can be realized.

During this time, considerable day-to-day coaching must take place, with emphasis on the behaviors that are cited in the criteria for each responsibility. This coaching will avoid unpleasant surprises at the first formal appraisal interview.

The time span for the first evaluation cycle will vary according to personnel policy and the informed decision of the department/division of nursing. A probationary period of three to six months is common for new employees. This same time frame can be used for the first evaluation cycle with all employees. Otherwise it may well be that the first cycle will be allowed to continue until the time designated for regular individual employee evaluation interviews.

Whatever the length of time decided upon, this entire phase allows the employee as well as the nurse manager to experience firsthand the initial use of both the job performance responsibilities and the performance criteria. During this time no changes should be made in the mutually agreed-upon job performance description (unless, of course, a grave error is noted or unforeseen job changes have been introduced).

ESTABLISHING MUTUAL GOALS AND OBJECTIVES

As the time approaches for the conclusion of Phase III, the nurse manager who is productivity oriented will be looking toward the performance evaluation interviews and planning for ways to combine management by objectives (MBO) with ROPEP.

As has been noted earlier, each employee should leave the interview with goals and objectives mutually agreed upon with the manager. Management by objectives, which is a results-oriented philosophy and system, is highly appropriate because it uses mutually established objectives, target dates, and evaluation of performance.

Figure 5-1 shows a combining of performance appraisal and management by objectives for productivity in nursing. It summarizes in six steps the functioning of an integrated MBO system that uses performance descriptions as the basis for performance evaluation in relation to individual personal objectives within the pattern of broad nursing department and organization goals.

The position used for the example is that of a nurse manager. Step I identifies some individuals and groups for whom the nurse manager performs key responsibilities—to patients, medical staff, nursing personnel, committee members, and hospital administration.

Step II gives examples of key performance responsibilities to those individuals; in this instance they are that the nurse manager will (1) assess quality of care to patients, (2) collaborate with the medical staff, (3) involve and evaluate nursing personnel, (4) utilize communication skills with committee members, and (5) manage the budget as a responsibility to hospital administration.

Step III delineates when performance is satisfactory based on predetermined performance criteria. The nurse manager's responsibility to the patient for assessing quality of care *is performed satisfactorily* when cri-

Figure 5-1 Combining Performance Appraisal and MBO for Nursing Productivity

Position: Nurse Manager

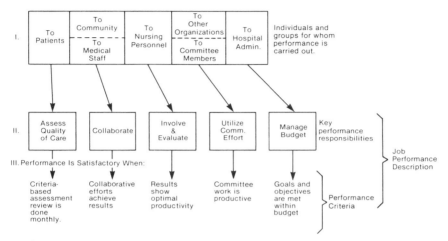

IV. Set specific goals and objectives

Set measurable, practical, achievable objectives that are mutually agreed upon.
Set target dates for completing objectives.

V. Perform as necessary to meet the set objectives and optimize productivity

VI. Review performance on the target dates

Measure and analyze performance and productivity results.
Set new and revised objectives.
Set new target dates.

Source: Adapted from *HELP with Performance Appraisal: A Results-Oriented Approach* by Joan M. Ganong and Warren L. Ganong with permission of W.L. Ganong Co., © 1981, p. 44.

teria-based assessment review is conducted monthly. Collaborative responsibilities with the medical staff are satisfactory when they achieve intended results. The responsibility to involve and evaluate nursing personnel is satisfactory when the results show optimal productivity. The responsibility to committee members to utilize communications skills is performed satisfactorily when the committee work is productive. Lastly, the nurse manager's responsibility to hospital administration to manage the budget is satisfactory when goals and objectives are met within the budget.

A job performance description thus must include the key performance responsibilities and the performance criteria. It may well include also the individuals and groups for whom performance is carried out, as in the example.

Step IV indicates the need for the nurse manager to set specific measurable, practical, and achievable goals and objectives in terms of the job performance responsibilities and criteria. These must be mutually agreed upon with the nurse manager's immediate superior (coordinator, assistant/associate director, nurse administrator), and must be in writing. Agreed target dates for completing those objectives also are set. Implied in all of these objectives are productivity standards that the nurse manager must meet to achieve optimal productivity on the job.

Step V is the time when the nurse manager performs as necessary in working toward meeting the objectives. Once again the hope here is to optimize productivity in the nurse manager's area of organizational responsibility.

Step VI is the review of the nurse manager's performance on the established target date. Each time this occurs, performance is measured and analyzed and productivity results are reviewed. New and revised objectives and target dates are set. At this point the cycle of Steps IV, V, and VI begins again and becomes a part of a continuing process for the nurse manager.

THE CONTINUING EVALUATION CYCLE, PHASE IV

Phase IV of ROPEP considers the continuing performance evaluation process once the initial developmental stages have been completed and the first work cycle and self-evaluation have occurred. At this point it is important to keep in mind what Peter Drucker emphasizes in his writings: that all one can measure is performance. And all one should measure is performance. One can measure a person's performance only against specific performance expectations.

As Phase IV begins, the nurse manager should refer once again to "Manager's Guide and Checklist" for the use of performance descriptions (Exhibit 4-3, supra). Employees will be doing their first self-evaluation utilizing the job performance description and whatever forms have been devised. Their entire focus should be on how well they feel they have met the responsibilities and standards of performance and behavioral criteria as stated in the job performance descriptions.

All individuals submit their own self-evaluation forms to the nurse manager at an agreed-upon date; some may elect to bring their forms with them rather than sending them in ahead of time. That is a personal decision between a nurse manager and an employee. In any event, the nurse manager should review the forms received in advance and be prepared for the first interview.

At the set dates and times the nurse manager conducts the first round of self-evaluation appraisal interviews. The focus is on identifying areas of mutual agreement on satisfactory and unsatisfactory performance. Next, mutual objectives and target dates for progress review are set. No employee should leave an appraisal interview without this very important step taking place.

It should be remembered that there is no necessity to find examples of unsatisfactory performance for every employee. For some, even when certain results are not fully satisfactory, emphasizing the positive results and behaviors may be the shortest route to motivating excellence in overall performance. In addition, skillful use of the MBO follow-through by manager and employee can reinforce positive results and help assure their continuity.

Following the appraisal interview, the employee goes back to the job very conscious of the need to work on the established objectives. The nurse manager's role during the follow-through work cycle is the day-to-day coaching coupled with observation of the employee and the results. A second round of appraisal interviews follows. This then becomes a cycle that involves work performance by each employee and the nurse manager, coupled with continuing as well as annual appraisal interviews.

Figure 5-2 portrays how the two management techniques of ROPEP and MBO help convert organizational purposes and goals into measurable achievements of the nursing division/department that fulfill the organizational mission. The sequence as shown on the diagram is as follows:

1. The Corporate Charter (Purpose or Mission Statement of the Organization)

Every organization exists for some purpose that is stated in its articles of incorporation or partnership. Hospitals frequently express their purpose as a statement of mission. This can be elaborated in the form of a number of specific goals.

2. Nursing Departmental Goals and Objectives

The nursing division or department exists to help achieve the purpose or mission of the organization. Thus nursing departmental goals and objectives must be: (1) consistent with the overall organizational purpose, (2)

Figure 5-2 ROPEP + MBO = Optimal Productivity: A Functional Diagram

1

The Corporate Charter
Mission
Purpose and Goals
of the Organization

2

Departmental
Goals and Objectives
Productivity Standards

3

Individual Employee
Performance Goals

Job Performance Description
• Purpose
• Responsibilities
• Performance Standards
  and Behavioral
  Criteria

Performance Objectives
• Related Activities
• Projects
• Special
  Assignments

4

Responsibilities I

IV Set Goals &
Objectives

II Job Segments

Perform V

ROPEP

Revisions

MBO

III Performance Standards

Review Progress VI

5

Results
Goal Achievement
Optimal Productivity

Source: Reprinted from *HELP with Performance Appraisal: A Results-Oriented Approach* by Joan M. Ganong and Warren L. Ganong with permission of W.L. Ganong Co., © 1981, p. 46.

identified in writing, and (3) departmentally distinctive as related to the division's (and each unit's) special function.

3. Job Purpose, Responsibilities, and Objectives

Within the nursing division/department, people work to help achieve its goals and objectives. Thus a job performance description identifies for each person the purpose, responsibilities, and measurable performance criteria to be met. Beyond normal responsibilities, however, are related activities, projects, and special assignments.

These are the short-term or longer term activities necessary to attain identified objectives that are steppingstones to goal achievement in the nursing department and the overall organization. For example: Doing the necessary work to implement the nursing process is essential to meeting Joint Commission on Accreditation of Hospitals (JCAH) accreditation standards for the benefit of hospital patients.

So it is with ROPEP, MBO, quality assurance, primary nursing, and similar nursing management techniques. When first introduced, all require a relatively short-term investment of concentrated effort from persons with a variety of other performance responsibilities. Once the initial implementation effort has been accomplished, the subsequent use and maintenance of such techniques becomes part of regular performance responsibilities.

4. The ROPEP-MBO Cycles

The next level shows both ROPEP and MBO as installed *management techniques* to be used by nurse managers in carrying out their *management functions* of planning, doing, and controlling. Thus a manager's performance appraisal interview involves not only a review of the nurse manager's results in carrying out his/her regular performance responsibilities but also progress and results on previously agreed-upon objectives.

5. Results

The hoped-for outcomes of this entire process are results that contribute to achievement of the purposes of the individual employee, the nursing division/department, and the organization. In hospitals and other health care entities, the expected beneficiaries are the patients/clients/consumers.

Exhibit 5-1 compares the cyclic processes of ROPEP and MBO with the "plan, do, and control" cycle of the management functions. The three cyclical processes just summarized are going on daily in one form or

Exhibit 5-1 Comparison of ROPEP, Management Functions, and MBO

The ROPEP Cycle	The Management Functions Cycle	The MBO Cycle
Identify Performance Responsibilities and Standards	PLAN	Set Goals and Objectives
Perform Job Segments	DO	Perform Necessary Work
Measure Performance against Standards and Criteria	CONTROL	Review Progress (Was the Objective Achieved on Time?)

Source: Reprinted from *HELP with Performance Appraisal: A Results-Oriented Approach* by John M. Ganong and Warren L. Ganong with permission of W.L. Ganong Co., © 1981, p. 87.

another for managers and employees alike. They are never ending. They are mutually dependent and supportive. They are this way because they are based upon proven principles and practices of participation and involvement of people working together toward common objectives.

THE PERFORMANCE APPRAISAL INTERVIEW

This section expands upon the important appraisal interview process presented in Chapter 4.

The appraisal interview is a one-to-one relationship between the employee and the nurse manager. When the interview is an occasion for helping an employee, the process may be thought of as a continuum of purpose that goes from interviewing, or the getting information from the individual, through advising or the giving of information or specific guidance, to counseling or the facilitating of personal discovery (Combs, Avila, & Purkey, 1971, p. 276).

Evaluation or appraisal is a continuing process. As has been pointed out, day-to-day coaching when properly carried out helps avoid surprises in the interview for both employee and nurse manager. Looked at in this way the appraisal interview can be said to be, "neither the beginning nor the end of anything. It is a middle step in a cycle that begins when an employee is hired to do a specific job and ends when he leaves it. If the other steps have been omitted or short-circuited, there is little hope for the appraisal interview" (Johnson, 1979, pp. 15–16).

The evaluation interview process consists of both structure and process. The structure within which the nurse manager operates consists of the welcome, moving through and keeping on track, agreeing on future goals and objectives, and bringing closure to the interview. In each of these pieces of structure a considerable amount of process takes place. Table 5-1 shows the relationship between structure and process.

Table 5-1 Appraisal Interview in Terms of Structure and Process

The Manager's Role

Structure	Process
1. Welcoming	1. Standing up Greeting Handshake Phrasing or wording Smiling, eye contact Seating arrangement
2. Moving through and keeping on track	2. Inviting employee to begin Keeping focus on job performance Listening passively Responding appropriately Agreeing where possible Using door openers Using summative feedback based on responsibilities and criteria Sharing "critical incidents"—anecdotal notes of specific instances of patterns of behavior Using items from "balance sheets" Using recognition and praise Clarifying areas of strength and those in need of strengthening
3. Agreeing on goals and objectives	3. Identifying specific challenges or need for changes in behavior Setting goals and objectives verbally and in writing Signing and dating evaluation form Using formative feedback if timely
4. Bringing closure	4. Sealing agreements Focusing on listening Speaking final words and phrases Summarizing Standing up Handshaking Smiling, eye contact

Welcoming

Welcoming the employee to an appraisal interview is an important part of the structure because it sets the stage or the tone for what is to follow. A welcome involves cordially greeting or receiving the person on arrival. It should not be done in an offhand manner. The process of welcoming usually includes such things as standing up and moving toward the employee, at the same time extending a verbal greeting and a warm handshake. Careful attention should be paid to eye contact and smiling.

All of this takes place fairly quickly and usually includes making certain that both parties have a comfortable seating arrangement. Wherever possible the two should be seated with no intervening barriers. Unless space is unusually cramped, there is no need for the manager to retreat behind a desk. More important than the seating arrangement itself, however, is the sincerity, openness, and warmth with which the employee is greeted and made to feel welcome.

It is important at this point that there be an assurance of privacy as well as comfort. Closing the door is really a way of saying that what is to occur is between the two persons and that confidentiality will be honored. Additional niceties can include the offering of coffee if that is a usual practice. Once again, the message in that offer implies that the manager wants the employee to feel welcome.

Moving Through and Keeping on Track

It is the responsibility of the nurse manager to assure that the reason for the interview is clarified at the outset. Once this is done the process takes over with an invitation to the employee to begin. This is important because with self-evaluation as the basis for a results-oriented job performance evaluation, the interview literally belongs to the employee.

The nurse manager needs to keep focusing on the overall purpose of the interview and to keep it on track. As the employee begins to share performance information, the manager moves to passive listening—a willingness to keep quiet usually is understood as reasonable evidence of interest and concern. Passive listening can be a potent tool for getting people to talk about what is on their mind. It gives them a sense of talking to someone who is willing to listen and who therefore acts as encouragement to keep going (Gordon, 1977, p. 55).

As the interview moves along the nurse manager responds appropriately, agreeing wherever possible with what the employee is saying. The use of "door openers" as an invitation to talk also can be useful: "Tell me more about that." "Can I be of any help?" "I'd be interested in your explanation of that."

The only purpose for collecting feedback information on performance is to do something with the material obtained. There are two classes of feedback decisions: (1) to increase or decrease the *likelihood* or *frequency* of a given performance (summative feedback) or (2) to correct, guide, or *modify the form* of that performance (formative feedback). The rules of summative feedback are well established and include being specific, providing feedback immediately after the behavior is observed, and being positive.

The three important dimensions of feedback are timing, clarity, and the degree of personalization that takes place while it is being given. Personalization also includes adequately informing the employee about what must be done to correct the behavior. This can be part of moving through the interview.

However, it should be remembered that the feedback given during the appraisal interview is primarily summative. It is not the time to work out a formative issue. Formative feedback, with corrective instruction, is best given *immediately before* the individual has an opportunity to use it (Tosti, 1980).

Keeping the interview on the track should include the sharing of specific critical incidents for which anecdotal notes may have been kept. These instances should show a pattern of behavior and not dwell on only one incident. This is especially true if the incident has been corrected and has never appeared again.

When patterns of unwanted behavior appear, that is evidence that the day-to-day coaching either has not taken place or has been ineffective. If feedback during the coaching has not taken place, the nurse manager must assume responsibility. Only the employee can assume the responsibility for not having changed the behavior to meet the criteria. It should be kept in mind that the appraisal interview should hold no surprises for either the nurse manager or the employee if the day-to-day coaching has been occurring.

A Balance-Sheet Approach

A balance-sheet approach is used by a nurse manager to identify both the positive and negative sides of an employee's behavior, an issue, a problem, or a proposed solution before looking at alternatives and taking action. A balance sheet, in the sense used here, is a statement of the assets and liabilities of an individual.

The nurse manager can prepare one by taking a sheet of paper and drawing a vertical line down the center. The left side stands for positive and the right side for negative factors. If this has been done before the interview on a criterion of particular importance in this individual's work, the sheet can serve as a visual means of showing whether the positives outweigh the negatives, or vice versa. The employee might be motivated to develop a personal balance sheet.

The balance sheet can be particularly helpful with an employee who is experiencing difficulty meeting behavioral criteria. However, it has other uses, such as helping decide which way to move on a particular issue or problem. It can assist both nurse manager and employee to decide upon what objectives to pursue.

Recognition and praise are an essential part of the appraisal interview process. A nurse manager's recognition of the employee's work is an acknowledgment of positive results in terms of performance responsibilities and criteria. Phrases that can be used include: "All of this indicates what a fine job you are doing in meeting this criterion." "You have made a splendid effort to meet the objectives we mutually agreed upon last time. Congratulations for a job well done." "You are really good at that."

Recognition is one of the needs of all people and as such it cries out to be met. Providing recognition is one of the least expensive of all of the motivators available to the nurse manager yet it is the one that is very much underused. It has a definite place in the appraisal interview. If recognition and earned praise have been given to the employee before the evaluation session, such feedback may not be new but it can act as a worthwhile reinforcer.

As the interview moves along the nurse manager needs to take time to clarify the areas of strengths and weaknesses that have been identified. These should be summarized verbally so they are clear to the employee. This also allows for correcting any possible misunderstandings in communication that may have occurred.

In some instances the employee may not have areas that need strengthening. It is a fallacy to believe that there always has to be something wrong with a person's performance. That kind of thinking has been encouraged by elaborate rating forms that sometimes emphasize weaknesses rather than strengths. If the performance does not require improvement, it may be necessary to look for challenges or special projects that the employee is interested in.

All too often an inordinate amount of time is spent on individuals whose performance does need improvement while those who are meeting all responsibilities and criteria satisfactorily are taken for granted.

Where results have been less than satisfactory, these have to be faced in the interview. The nurse manager must seek mutual understanding and agreement with the evidence of unsatisfactory results. Where there is disagreement, the nurse manager must make it clear what particular behaviors are unsatisfactory but must avoid personality traits or isolated incidents. A balance-sheet approach also can be helpful in this situation.

Agreeing on Goals and Objectives

To keep the interview on the track it is necesary to identify either the specific challenges or the need for changes in behavior that the employee can work on in the near future. If at all possible, it should be the employee who suggests what to do about it. After all, if improvement in behavior is to occur it has to come through the individual's own efforts.

Once the areas have been identified, specific goals and objectives should be discussed verbally and eventually put into writing. Exhibit 5-2 demonstrates how this can be done using an objectives work sheet approach. No employees should leave a performance appraisal interview without knowing what the nurse manager expects of them and what they should expect of themselves. The goals and objectives should delineate clearly what is to be accomplished, how soon, who will help, what each person will do, how soon that will be done.

The goal is stated simply as an overall purpose or an aim, such as "to improve my nursing care plans" or "to work more effectively with my colleagues" or "to obtain the required amount of inservice education programs dealing with patient assessment." The objectives, however, should be task-oriented statements of results to be achieved in order to reach the overall goal. Objectives must be measurable, practical, and achievable. For example, a primary nurse might write: "Will complete or update daily a nursing care plan for all assigned patients beginning (date) and to be evaluated by (target date)."

The objectives should be few in number, particularly since some employees may be able to work on only one at a time. The objectives need to be jointly developed and mutually agreed upon by both the nurse manager and the employee. The goals and objectives should be in writing, signed by the nurse manager and the employee, and should be dated.

Bringing Closure

As the appraisal interview begins to draw to a close, there is a need for sealing the oral and written agreements on what has occurred and what is to take place. Once again the nurse manager should focus on listening,

Exhibit 5-2 Objectives Work Sheet

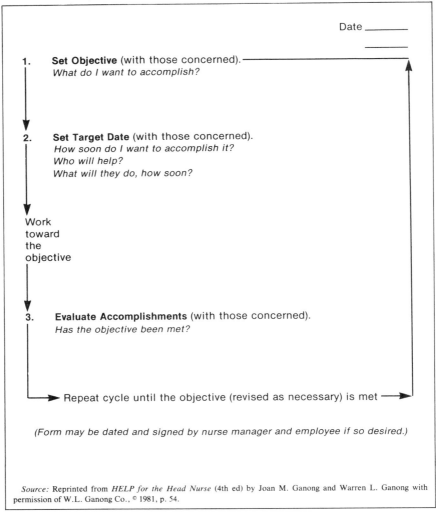

Date _____
_____

1.   **Set Objective** (with those concerned). ————————————
     What do I want to accomplish?

2.   **Set Target Date** (with those concerned).
     How soon do I want to accomplish it?
     Who will help?
     What will they do, how soon?

Work
toward
the
objective

3.   **Evaluate Accomplishments** (with those concerned).
     Has the objective been met?

Repeat cycle until the objective (revised as necessary) is met

(Form may be dated and signed by nurse manager and employee if so desired.)

Source: Reprinted from *HELP for the Head Nurse* (4th ed) by Joan M. Ganong and Warren L. Ganong with permission of W.L. Ganong Co., © 1981, p. 54.

primarily active listening, using the final words and phrases that will summarize the results of the session.

This should be done briefly and should lead to the manager's bringing the interview to a close by standing up and extending a hand for a handshake. A smile, eye contact, and words of encouragement can give the employee a feeling that there is something positive to look forward to.

Additional appraisal interviewing guidelines for the nurse manager are included in chapters 4 and 7.

SIMPLICITY THE BEST SYSTEM

This chapter has dealt with the payoff final two phases of the results-oriented performance appraisal program—namely, the first evaluation cycle and the continuing evaluation cycle. This is when the nurse manager's developmental efforts and coaching expertise become evident through employee behavior and performance results. This also is when the output side of the productivity formula can provide increasing satisfaction to the nurse manager in terms of the quality and costs of patient care.

Users of ROPEP will do well to recall that it is one of the hybrid performance appraisal systems that incorporate features of several appraisal approaches and the increased use of MBO. McGregor (1957) suggested that this MBO approach to appraisal has the advantages of:

1. redefining the manager's role to that of helper rather than judge,
2. increasing subordinate acceptance, since the emphasis is on performance rather than personality,
3. Shifting the orientation toward future actions instead of past behavior.

ROPEP can produce these and related benefits for those who use it well.

Do ROPEP's four phases seem complicated or too time consuming? They need not be. In fact, the appraisal program should be kept as simple as possible while adhering to sound principles. The simplest things often are the most profound—and the most productive.

For example, *The One Minute Manager* (Blanchard & Johnson, 1982) is a deceptively simple and captivating summary of some profound management practices. The focus is on one minute goal setting, one minute praisings, and one minute reprimands. Careful readers will quickly recognize the way these skillful authors have captured the essence of valuable behavioral theory so that it can be readily understood and used. Example: "Catch someone doing something right."

The authors also recognize that "one minute management" will work only if certain systems are built into the organization.

"The first is an accountability system, so that people in the organization are clear on what they are asked to do. The second is a data system. Companies have all sorts of information, but very little of it is helpful to managing individuals. So we're helping them set up data systems tied to goals of job performance.

"The third system is feedback—and getting it to employees as often as possible. A once-a-year performance evaluation is not going to do the job. The fourth system is recognition. The accountability and data systems help in the goal setting, and the feedback and recognition systems get into the praising and reprimands." (Making Brevity, 1983)

This reinforces the earlier emphasis here on performance appraisal as just one element (but an important one) of the total management system. The next chapter shows how the performance appraisal program can be integrated with another system element, a career ladder program.

For Discussion Purposes

By this time the task force has involved a large number of people in the review, and possible redesign, of the nursing department performance appraisal program. There is a better appreciation of how performance appraisal relates to other nursing and hospital management techniques and practices. There is a growing realization, among all levels of nursing department personnel, of how an effectively administered criteria-based performance appraisal plan will influence productivity and quality assurance.

Give your understanding of how this can be made to happen.

NOTES

Blanchard, K., & Johnson, S. *The one minute manager*. New York: William Morrow & Company, Inc., 1982.

Combs, A.W.; Avila, D.L.; & Purkey, W.W. *Helping relationships: Basic concepts for the helping professions*. Boston: Allyn & Bacon, Inc., 1971.

Drucker, P. *Management: Tasks, responsibilities, practices*. New York: Harper & Row, Publishers, Inc., 1974.

Ganong, J.M., & Ganong, W.L. *HELP for the head nurse (4th ed.)*. Chapel Hill, N.C.: W.L. Ganong Co., 1981. (a)

Ganong, J.M., & Ganong, W.L. *HELP with performance appraisal: A results-oriented approach*. Chapel Hill, N.C.: W.L. Ganong Co., 1981. (b)

Gordon, T. *Leadership effectiveness training, L.E.T.* New York: Peter H. Wyden, Inc., 1977.

Johnson, R.G. *The appraisal interview guide*. New York: AMACOM, 1979.

Making brevity the soul of management. *Management Review*, March 1983, *72*(3), 4.

McGregor, D. "An uneasy look at performance appraised." Harvard Business Review, 1957, 35(3), 89–94.

Tosti, D. The sequential feedback model for performance assessment. In J.W. Springer (Ed.), *Job performance standards and measures* (Paper No. 4, ASTD Research Series). Madison, Wis.: American Society for Training and Development, 1980.

Chapter 6

Career Ladders: Aid to Productivity

PERSPECTIVES ON CAREER MANAGEMENT

Career ladders for nurses have been much talked about over the years. Only since the early 1970s has that interest been translated into significant action. Even now, the term "career ladder" sometimes is used as though it were synonymous with "clinical ladder."

A career ladder program is defined as a viable system for providing selective career options with progression of responsibility and earnings on three main tracks in nursing—managerial, educational, and clinical—within a single health care agency. Research can be included as a fourth track, shown in Figure 6-2 as cutting across the other three pathways. The program uses agency-developed (within the hospital or facility) criteria for defining the steps on each track, the necessary continuing education and training, and related qualifying procedures. It also provides an opportunity to move from one track to another (Ganong, 1982a).

(A few hospitals include additional professional development tracks for bedside nurses as described in Appendix I on the New England Medical Center.)

Introducing career ladders is the logical follow-through for nursing departments that have invested in an up-to-date, results-oriented performance appraisal technique as part of the organization's human resources management program. In fact, job performance descriptions should be so written that they serve the purposes of both performance appraisal and career ladders. This is the most economical approach and serves well the combined goals for both productivity and quality assurance.

Too often a great deal of time and expense is devoted to developing presumed scientific approaches designed with the best of intentions for accuracy and fairness. Such efforts sometimes reflect a needless rigidity in the wage and salary administration program and at other times indicate the misguided counsel of advisers or consultants.

The authors call it "spending megabucks with a nickel-and-dime approach to individual take-home pay." They espouse a system that recognizes the reality of a variety of factors' influencing wages (see Chapter 1) and the fact that the performance appraisal system sometimes is manipulated in the interest of cost control.

Instead, the authors prefer an appraisal system that is not directly related to the wage and salary system but is based on measurable performance standards built into the job performance descriptions with criteria for both quality and quantity of results. This should be combined with an institutional point of view that nurses deserve top dollar if they are "satisfactory" (worth keeping) because they meet the performance standards and should be paid at least in the upper half of the appropriate salary range. If they are unsatisfactory in significant aspects of performance and are not retrainable, then they may be transferred or released (Ganong & Ganong, 1982a).

This chapter provides guidance in designing and initiating a career ladder program. The timeliness of the subject is emphasized by the following introduction to an information survey report in *RN* magazine:

> Looking for a specialty where jobs will go begging? Want to stay as marketable as possible? Check this picture of nursing only five years down the road. There will be:
>
> - Two and a half times more hospice units than now,
> - Double the number of hospital-based home care services,
> - Explosive growth in short stay, ambulatory, rehab, and oncology units,
> - Ten percent *fewer* psych openings,
> - A dramatic increase in demand for specialty certification. (Gulack, 1983, p. 35)

The article includes graphic projections on the changing profile of the nation's hospitals between 1982 and 1987. The 1987 predictions anticipate rapid growth in many of the 37 specialty services that offer an alternative to the traditional acute care approach. Figure 6-1 shows the growth expected in R.N. positions for 12 of those services between 1982 and 1987.

HISTORICAL OVERVIEW

In years past, most nurses did not design career plans. Indeed, most of the registered nurses in the United States were not career oriented. They

Figure 6-1 Shifting Prospects at the Traditional Core

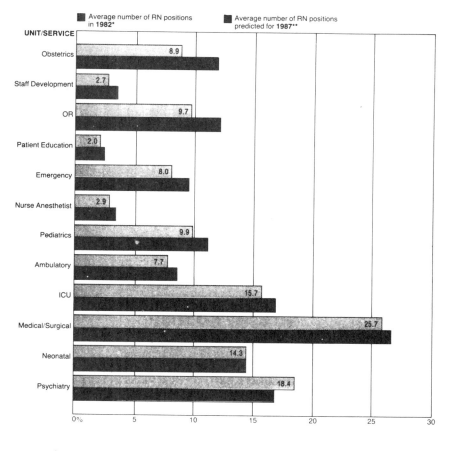

■ Average number of RN positions in **1982***   ■ Average number of RN positions predicted for **1987****

*Calculated on the basis of all respondents who reported data concerning 1982, regardless of whether they made predictions concerning 1987
**Calculated on the basis of all respondents who made predictions concerning 1987, regardless of whether they reported data concerning 1982

Source: Reprinted from "The Main Chance" by R. Gulack with permission of *RN,* March 1983, *46*(3), 38, © 1983.

took a nursing job when they graduated from nursing school. For some, this led to a lifetime commitment to a single hospital. Some who married combined homemaking with working; others gave up nursing. Still others went wherever the prospects looked best or moved with husbands as the needs of their employment dictated. Jobs always were available. Much of the job activity was random, with minimal career planning in mind. Sometimes, nurses who remained single or became single because of death of a spouse or divorce developed a conscious effort to carve out a career in the field.

Nurses worked as staff nurses, head nurses or as supervisors—and some as inservice educators or as school faculty members—with some of them eventually moving on to top-level nursing jobs. Most of these positions were in hospitals or public health agencies. There was little cross-over between education and "service." In any event the focus was more on nursing as a job than as a career. As vacancies occurred staff nurses were promoted to head nurses and so on up the hierarchy.

"Too often in the past, changed roles in nursing practice have been hampered by our traditional 'promotion' system that has tended to draw practitioners away from the patient by advancing them to positions where managerial functions quickly replace care procedures." (Lysaught, 1974)

Following World War II, nurses returning to civilian life often took advantage of the GI Bill and went on for higher education, a trend that expanded substantially in the 1950s and beyond. More baccalaureate programs emerged. The number of hospitals and beds increased dramatically. Licensed practical nurses as well as nurse aides appeared on the scene. Also in the 1950s the associate degree nurse came into being, and with this the emerging new patterns of preparing nurses spread across the country like spilled paint.

With all of this diversity of preparation, no clear-cut career planning was in evidence. Hospitals, which continue to be the employers of the greatest percentage of registered nurses, gave little attention to a career ladder that would permit them to plan a career in a single organization. To advance at all in such hospitals, nurses had to leave the bedside and move into nursing supervision.

> Examination of the organization and structure of traditional nursing services leads to the conclusion that (1) failure to formally recognize in practice through a ladder for clinical advancement and (2) failure to provide an environment which enables nurses to grow in competence may be omissions that contribute to lack of incentive to either achieve an advanced level of competence in practice or to pursue careers at the bedside. (Zimmer, 1972)

National Study Recommendations

In *An Abstract for Action* published as a report of the National Commission for the Study of Nursing and Nursing Education, Lysaught (1970) points out the need to retain nurses in practice, reduce turnover, and provide reasonable and needed incentives for them to continue in direct care activities. This led to the study's Recommendation #3 that:

> Health management administrators and clinical directors of nursing service build on current improvements in starting salaries to create a strong reward system for remaining in clinical practice by developing schedules of substantially increasing salary levels for experienced nurses functioning in advanced capacities . . .

and Recommendation #4 that:

> Personnel policies in all health care facilities should be so designed that they (a) Differentiate levels of responsibility in accord with the concepts of staff nurse, clinical nurse, and master clinician with appropriate intermediate grades. These levels should be designed according to the content of the position and the clinical proficiency required for competent performance; (b) Provide for promotion granted on the basis of acquisition of the knowledge and demonstrated competence to perform in a given position (p. 134).

Those recommendations were developed after a finding that most promotional opportunities were based on time in grade or on formal educational achievements. Thus there was recognition for longevity and additional course work but not necessarily for demonstrated knowledge and competence in nursing practice attained through informal education, self-study, or experience.

As the medical and health technologies boomed in the 1970s there was an ever-increasing need to recruit and retain clinically competent registered nurses in hospitals. Clinical advancement programs began to appear. Many of these were based on the concept that:

> nursing like other professions is practiced at several levels of skill and competence, and that clinical nurses should be rewarded according to their levels of expertise. . . . The clinical advancement program at Indiana University Hospital affirms that the primary goal of nursing is care delivery to patients and their families with the professional practice model. The program has been in effect for two years. A preliminary assessment suggests that it has successfully motivated both new and experienced nurses, and has had far-reaching and positive effects throughout the entire nursing organization. . . . probably the most positive

outcome of the clinical advancement program is that it validates and exemplifies nursing service's commitment to reward clinical expertise. (Knox, 1980, 29–33)

The Career Ladder Needed

The need for a clinical promotion ladder within a single institution is critical. At the same time, the practice of nursing requires knowledgeable and skillful leadership and management. Therefore, a need also exists to provide definite promotional ladders for nurses in management, education, staff development, and research.

An example of a career ladder program is the one at the Cincinnati General Hospital, University of Cincinnati Medical Center. That program combines on-the-job training with paid tuition to local schools of nursing, and tutoring, to provide career mobility for its employees. It abolishes the dead-end aspects of jobs in the nursing department.

Another example of a successful career ladder program with a broad approach beyond just the clinical is the REAP (Rex Employee Advancement Program) at Rex Hospital, Raleigh, N.C. (Ganong & Ganong, 1980, pp. 352–364). The Rex Hospital program recognizes that the facility's survival and well-being are dependent upon those who build their careers there. This program, which went into effect July 29, 1974, has the following features and benefits.

1. Identifies for *all* nursing service employees the pathways to earned promotions and merited increases in pay.
2. Provides both clinical and managerial promotional channels for qualified personnel beyond the present R.N. practitioner level.
3. Establishes standards of performance and a performance review plan for all job levels.
4. Provides additional promotional steps within specific job categories (N.A., R.N., L.P.N., W.S.).
5. Permits merit pay increases within job categories as promotions are earned from one step to another, based upon ability to satisfactorily perform additional tasks.
6. Assures qualified persons for nursing service positions.
7. Permits staffing each unit with the minimum number of qualified personnel with a resultant saving in wage costs.
8. Requires that persons who qualify for higher job levels be able to perform all tasks identified for lower paid job levels and to

actually perform those tasks when staffing emergencies occur. (Ganong & Ganong, 1980, pp. 356–357)

The introduction of a career ladder program requires the support and interest of more than just the Department of Nursing. It requires, as pointed out in the 1981 follow-up on the recommendations of the National Commission for the Study of Nursing and Nursing Education, "the support and commitment of health administrators and physicians as well as the best efforts of the nursing profession. . . . A start has been made; discernible progress can be documented over the past decade. But in 1980 we still have far to go" (Lysaught, 1981, p. 147).

The National Commission Study

The seriousness of the "nursing shortage" of the 1970s led to the unique multidisciplinary effort in the form of a National Commission on Nursing (NCN) that began its work in September 1980. It was charged with developing and implementing action plans for the future of nursing. Its full charge was broad:

- Analyze the internal and external forces that influence the environment of nurses at work.
- Identify the effects of professional nursing issues on nursing practice in health care agencies.
- Assess the professional characteristics of nurses in relation to the organizational structure of health care agencies.
- Explore the motivation and incentives for nursing education and nursing practice.
- Analyze the relationship among education, nursing practice, and professional interaction in the health care agency.
- Develop a platform of issues to be dealt with in the commission activities.
- Plan methods to enhance the professional status and top management role of the nurse through:
  - research to define status and role.
  - publication of information to describe or explain status and role in relationship to health care.
  - demonstration projects to provide models for problem resolution, development, and reshaping of relationships and structures in health care agencies. (NCN, 1981)

This panel consisted of 30 leaders in nursing, hospital management, medicine, government, academia, and business, with Marjorie Beyers, R.N., Ph.D., as director.

This independent commission was sponsored jointly by The American Hospital Association, the Hospital Research and Educational Trust, and the American Hospital Supply Corporation. The sponsorship alone signifies the concern of the hospital industry for the role that nursing would assume through the coming decades.

The commission reports that the most frequently mentioned factors promoting job satisfaction for nurses are salaries and benefits, staffing and scheduling, working conditions, and career opportunities (NCN, 1981, pp. 28–29). The report calls for institutions to examine their management practices as well as to listen to their staff nurses and to work toward comprehensive retention programs.

"Staffing shortages which threaten the economic status of hospitals are impelling these institutions to initiate employment practices supportive of nurses in new and less subservient roles" (Steck, 1981). One thing that the career ladder does when instituted in a hospital is break with tradition. It places more emphasis on performance than on tenure. It relates salary increases to predetermined performance criteria. It also offers nurses career options not available to them before.

Some nurses may find that their work is evaluated more systematically, and for a time that may prove to be unsettling. Therefore, hospitals implementing a major change such as the nursing career ladder program must be prepared to deal with negative as well as positive reactions (Alt, Bates, Gilmore, Houston, & Stoner, 1980).

In predictions for the 1990s, Coogan (1981) expects that the nurses' new status will show up in their wallets and working conditions. Specifically, Coogan anticipates standardized education levels, specialization career ladders, and, in the face of a continuing personnel shortage, pay scales that reward nurses who advance. Coogan also predicts that the trend for required continuing education will become a key part of a career ladder program for everyone. If these predictions are to be realized in the 1990s, much work will have to be done in the rest of the 1980s to provide full-fledged career ladders for registered nurses.

INITIATING AND DEVELOPING CAREER LADDERS

A career ladder program in nursing is defined at the beginning of this chapter. A model for career ladders—the multiple track careers concept—is shown in Figure 6-2.

Figure 6-2 A Model for Career Ladders in Nursing

The Career Pathways

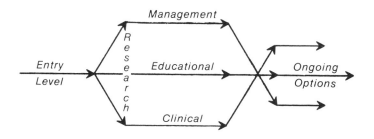

The Career Ladders

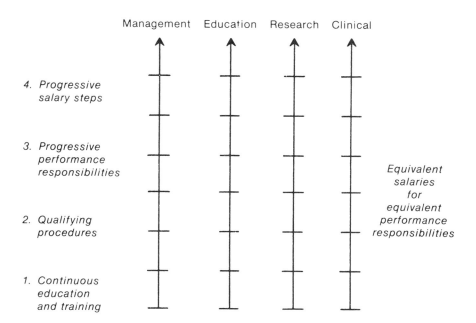

Source: Reprinted from *HELP with Wide-Track Careers in Nursing* by Joan M. Ganong and Warren L. Ganong with permission of W.L. Ganong Co., © 1977, p. 6.

First are the three main career pathways (clinical, educational, management), with opportunities for nurses to move from one track to another—including research, when that is a feasible option, cutting across the other tracks.

The concept also is presented as four career ladders with an ascending scale of progressive salary steps. The rungs represent, at each level, equivalent salaries for equivalent performance responsibilities. (Such salary scales commonly are set by job and salary evaluation. For a discussion of the drawbacks of this technique and an explanation of another innovative method, see Jaques, 1979.)

It should be noted that the nurses' salary progression depends on their having prepared themselves for additional responsibilities through a qualifying procedure based in part on in-house availability of suitable education and training programs.

Actual salary adjustments occur in the career ladder program when the prepared person has been promoted into a higher level job classification. This means having an expanded number of job classifications on all four tracks. At Rex Hospital (noted earlier) the levels of progression on the clinical track are set up as in Exhibit 6-1.

An increasing number of hospitals and other health care organizations provide specific career opportunities that justify showing research as one of four main tracks open to qualified nurses, especially when career progress is being considered broadly in an interagency or multihospital system context.

Exhibit 6-1 Progression Levels on Clinical Track

N.A. I N.A. II N.A. III P.N. L.P.N. I L.P.N. II L.P.N. III G.N. R.N. I R.N. II R.N. III R.N. IV	Each of these performance levels on the clinical track was selected and defined to provide a meaningful career ladder. The number of steps from N.A. I through R.N. IV is affected in part by a pragmatic approach as to how they will fit within the agencywide wage and salary system.

Source: Reprinted from *HELP with Wide-Track Careers in Nursing* by Joan M. Ganong and Warren L. Ganong with permission of W.L. Ganong Co., © 1977, p. 6.

However, the career ladder program is presented here as an intraagency management technique because it was developed to cope with some recognized problems in hospitals that impinge upon the three major responsibilities of nurse managers—clinical, operational, and human resources management (Ganong & Ganong, 1980). Intraagency problems that nurse managers face include the need to:

1. reduce the high rate of turnover among nurses
2. recruit nursing personnel who have long-term employment potential
3. offer meaningful inducements to retain the best employees
4. provide job progression opportunities related to pay increases for all nursing personnel but especially for those who provide direct bedside care and services to patients
5. view nursing as a process rather than as a series of unrelated tasks
6. utilize patient care modalities based on the nursing process in a way that wins the respect of nurses, other health professionals, and patients
7. cope with the identity problem caused by the American Nursing Association's role as a labor union for nurses while being the only professional organization that speaks for nursing through its lobbying efforts in Washington and in numerous states
8. maintain the status and clout necessary in administrative councils justified by the scope of the Nursing Department's patient care, legal, and physical responsibilities on a 24-hour basis
9. respond to the contentions and restraints growing out of the escalating cost containment crunch
10. justify to hospital administration and governing bodies the annual budgets that reflect the foregoing problems
11. cope with the increasing emphasis on competition being fostered in the health care industry as a whole
12. adjust to the proliferation of certification, registration, licensure, and employment regulations and changes affecting health care personnel at all levels
13. deal with the promulgations and influence of the many associations representing the varied groups of employees.

A multiple-track career program is one way of facing the facts of life in today's health care workworld. It builds upon available assets and strengths while at the same time being fully pragmatic and facing the necessity for rigid cost control. It is sufficiently idealistic and rationally realistic to incorporate the tested tenets of humanistic psychology, sound organizational development, and motivational management.

Career mobility is an idea whose time certainly has come. The multiple-track concept offers more than mobility of nurses from job to job, from one health care agency to another, from city to city, and from state to state. It provides mobility in the sense of a carefully defined plan for career progress within an individual hospital or related organization. This meets the needs of institutional nursing personnel, who traditionally have lacked meaningful career options that are clearly identified and supported by well-structured qualifying programs integrated with progressive wage and salary policies.

Purposes and Objectives

The purpose of a multiple-track career program is to obtain the maximum possible return on an ever-growing investment in human resources. Its objectives are to:

1. justify the initial set-up cost of beginning a multiple-track career program
2. facilitate and coordinate the program performance plan steps necessary for implementation
3. relate and integrate the concepts of multiple-track careers within a single agency's existing management philosophy, practices, and techniques
4. prepare job performance descriptions, a performance evaluation plan, and practical career ladders with attendant salary scales
5. provide earning opportunities commensurate with responsibilities along all four tracks—management, educational, research, and clinical
6. control and evaluate the effectiveness of a multitrack career program as a continuing management technique.

The introduction of a career ladder program proceeds most smoothly when the hospital provides a reasonably sophisticated administrative support system, characterized by the following concepts, principles, and practices:

1. Every hospital employee affects patient care, its quality, and its cost.
2. Organizational accountability is dependent upon each employee's sense of accountability to self.
3. Personal responsibility is considered an inherent component of each person's sense of self-worth, not as something delegated from above.

4. Motivation is a personal matter; it comes from within.
5. Managers assist each person's self-motivation by creating a working environment that helps all employees meet their needs while contributing to organizational goals.
6. The nature of superior/subordinate daily relationships affects, and is affected by, each person's level of need satisfaction (survival, security, social, status, self-actualization).
7. Organization charts are used effectively in communicating and clarifying the formal organizational structure, relationships, and fiscal responsibility.
8. The structure of organization is adaptive rather than monolithic; different units or departments may have their own unique ways of organizing and functioning to meet the needs of patients and personnel.
9. Fair labor practices require *unequal* (differing kinds of) treatment of employees, based upon their individual needs and problems.
10. Decision-making authority is held by personnel at every level, especially by those closest to the patients (within legal, professional, and organizational guidelines).
11. Problem solving is facilitated horizontally and vertically throughout the organization—the matrix model.
12. Power and communication centers are varied and dispersed—the homeostatic biological model.
13. The structure demands the use of motive force and innovative action from the greatest possible number of persons.
14. Intradepartmental coordination and control require minimal attention but are effective through use of the management process at all levels.
15. Widespread nurse manager involvement in utilizing the management functions and techniques at all levels permits meeting current objectives while identifying and planning future goals for all three responsibilities—management of patient care, department operations, and human resources.
16. Policy manuals are up to date and serve as guidelines to action.
17. Procedure manuals provide suitable operating instructions and indicate when variations from practice are unsafe, illegal, or otherwise not permissible.
18. Unit profiles define each patient care unit, including a description of the nursing care modality.
19. Unit and departmental budgetary planning and control are fully decentralized as a year-round function; budgets are based on goals and objectives related to patient care programs.

20. Suitable staff support personnel (for such activities as nurse recruiting, scheduling, budgeting, systems analysis, procedures development, methods improvement, staff development, quality assurance,
top-level clinical assistance, research, long-range planning) are provided for the nurse managers either within the nursing department
or interdepartmentally, as appropriate within the specific agency.
(Ganong & Ganong, 1982b, pp. 10–12)

Such beliefs and practices as these facilitate the introduction of a career
ladder program. In any event, planning for career ladders must take into
account the hospital's management philosophy, practices, and techniques,
especially as they affect human resources management, wage and salary
administration, fiscal accountability, and patient care modalities.

Where to Begin?

In anything, people always have to begin from where they are. So
initiation of this career ladder program begins by identifying where people
are—as persons, as a department, as a hospital. This means taking inventory. An individual who is director of nursing, already has a good idea of
what the inventory will show. Yet others in the department and hospital,
taking the same inventory, will provide other views. At the beginning, it
thus is important to include others in the approach to career ladders.

First is the superior. It is helpful to remember the dictum: "Never let
your boss be surprised." Others then are included; the superior may
suggest one or two persons. It is worthwhile considering someone from
the personnel department, staff development, key nurse managers, and
inservice education. It may be appropriate to have them act as a career
ladder task force. All nurse managers should be informed of what is being
done and should be involved as pertinent. Successful change—especially
innovative change—requires the involvement of those who will be affected
by it.

The task force should be assigned to research the career ladder concept;
members should be provided with copies of suitable guidebooks (Ganong
& Ganong, 1982b), invited to explore the references in the literature, and
investigate what others have done.

Before the task force recommends a course of action, the nurse manager
should be sure it provides the inventory it has developed on "Where we
are—as nurses, a department, a hospital." This is important because of
the impact of a career ladder program (even the fact of its being explored)
on the entire organization. No significant program should be introduced
without careful planning to consider its effect on other elements of the

organizational structure, interrelationships, policies, procedures, and practices. Hence the wisdom of the initial inventory. (See Chapter 3, particularly Table 3-2, for the Nursing Organization Inventory Checklist and a discussion of each item.)

Preparing for Action

The successful completion of the inventory checklist will involve substantial numbers of people both in and outside of the nursing department. Those outside who need to participate include persons with such titles as personnel director, wage and salary administrator, human resources director, associate administrator, hospital administrator, controller, management engineering director, hospital planner, labor relations attorney, and budgetary coordinator.

The timing and extent of the involvement of such persons depends largely upon the hospital's organizational situation, current priorities, and resources available within the nursing department itself.

The inventory checklist should be completed just as thoroughly as possible by the nursing management group itself before seeking assistance from others outside the department. The benefits of doing so are many:

1. It provides a useful evaluation of the knowledgeability of the members of the group regarding the listed items that influence department operation.
2. The process of completing the inventory will suggest the questions that need to be asked.

Once these questions have been formulated, the patient care administrator (nursing director) can take them to the hospital administrator (executive director, vice president) for suggestions as how best to find the answers. This should be done with an explanation of the reasons for the questions. Even if the administrator can answer them, it is better that they be pursued with the appropriate department heads or staff persons as a means of beginning to involve them in the exploratory stages of a career ladder program.

The particular strategy to be used is best identified by those in nursing who are most familiar with the hospital personnel as long as the principles of early involvement and constructive participation are kept in mind. This approach presupposes that the nursing management group has a clear understanding of career ladder concepts and has defined the goals and objectives for such a program.

The introduction of a career ladder program necessitates a variety of changes in the hospital's policies and practices. Most of the changes are predictable and can be planned so that they create a minimum of surprises or discomfort. However, some individuals may feel the change process can threaten the satisfying of their needs so it can cause unforeseen reactions. These deserve to be recognized for what they are and be dealt with in a way that relieves the anxiety of individuals and permits them to contribute constructively to the change process.

Clarifying the Goal

The primary purpose of a career ladder program in hospital nursing is to provide opportunities for qualified individuals to progress along one or more career tracks of their choice. The steps in each track must be defined carefully. Knowledge, skill, and performance requirements have to be developed for each level of each ladder. Those who aspire to higher levels then can identify what they must know and be able to do to qualify for the better positions as vacancies occur.

Job descriptions, especially in connection with career ladders, provide a management tool for defining performance levels. A performance level is a specified degree of knowledge, competency, and experience required to carry out a particular position satisfactorily; it also clearly delineates the differences between the performance characteristics of one job classification and another.

Knowledge is the first factor necessary for satisfactory performance in every position. The kinds and degree of knowledge vary widely from job to job but satisfactory performance always is dependent upon an understanding of the position's purpose and the reasons for the what and how of the job function.

The second factor is competency or skill, both mental and manual. Skill is acquired by practicing the right method. Satisfactory performance is dependent upon proficiency in doing.

The third factor influencing the definition of performance level is experience. Higher job levels commonly require longer experience (length of service) in lower level work categories. When such experience is meaningful (and is combined with continuing education), it provides the breadth and depth of knowledge and expertise required for satisfactory performance in the higher level job. To that extent, recognition of length of service in the wage and salary plan has validity.

Policies and Procedures

Planning for career ladders gives rise to many questions that suggest the need for developing policies and procedures to guide implementation of the program. Nurse managers should begin to accumulate the questions (that will need answering) as they occur to themselves and to others during the many months of program development work. Maintaining a list of questions will help to shape the final design of the career ladder program. Then, when development efforts are nearly complete, the material will be in hand for writing a meaningful set of policies and procedures.

In any event, the eventual career ladder policy and procedure guidelines will reflect many existing nursing department and hospital policies. This is one of the reasons for compiling the nursing organization inventory. Completion of that inventory puts nurse managers in a better position to judge the extent to which existing policies and procedures must be followed carefully, modified, expanded, or supplemented to permit an effective career ladder program. Appendixes H and I at the end of the book provide examples of policy development.

BENEFITS FROM DEVELOPING A PROGRAM

The planning and development of a career ladder program provides a number of benefits. It provides a boost in morale as many people get involved. They work together toward a meaningful goal. They contribute, their ideas are listened to. Naturally they feel good. They are meeting some of their basic human needs.

Next is role clarification. Supervisors and subordinates jointly develop the performance descriptions. Mutual expectations are clarified. Then there are the methods improvement possibilities. Detailed listing of nursing procedures and activities stimulates questioning. "Take the corners off your thinking" and ideas for improvements flow naturally. The four steps of work simplification should be used: eliminate, combine, change sequence, simplify.

Planning for career ladders encourages a broad view of nursing in toto. It permits nurse managers to develop their own *Framework for Nursing Management* (See Figure 1-1, Chapter 1). Help with wage and salary administration is another benefit. The pay levels criteria establish bona fide career steps, each one with more demanding qualifications than the previous one, providing valid data for wage and salary progression. Dollar scales can be directly related to measurable performance requirements.

Similarly, there is built-in merit progression. The added ladder steps provide regular opportunities for employees in each job category to move ahead and into higher paid classifications. This obviates the need for a separate, often ill-fated (as noted earlier), "merit rating" plan.

TURNOVER, CAREER LADDERS, PRODUCTIVITY

To assure some measure of continuity of patient care, a certain amount of stability is necessary among the registered nurses on any unit. A major problem that plagues hospitals is nurse turnover. Price and Mueller (1981, p. 2) define turnover as the voluntary separation of an individual from an organization. From the perspective of the hospital, Price and Mueller cite three reasons for the importance of turnover.

One reason is that it seriously complicates providing quality care for patients. Nurses are critically important since they are the most highly trained professionals who are continually present over a 24-hour period each day, every day. Clearly, nursing turnover threatens the hospital's effectiveness and adds to its expense. If institutions want to maintain standards of patient care and improve productivity they must reduce nursing turnover significantly.

A second reason is the need for hospitals to establish alternate career structures for nurses. The traditional hierarchical structure consists mostly of administrative occupations. Once again this emphasizes the need for a focus on staff nurses who primarily are in a professional occupation. "Staff nurses who render direct patient care need to have more control over their own work. This is a logical first step in promoting job satisfaction as well as reducing turnover and promoting the professionalization of nursing." (Alexander, Weisman, & Chase, 1982)

Some hospitals with high turnover have been reluctant to establish alternate career paths because of the expense. However, the high cost of turnover itself is a problem. Wolf (1981) cites the cost to replace one R.N. as $2,500 to $3,000, including orientation, preemployment physicals, processing expenses, overtime for those who fill in during a vacancy, or registry fees to fill the vacant positions. This reluctance to consider alternative approaches is likely to result in serious long-term problems.

A third reason for the importance of turnover is that the geographical maldistribution of nurses across the country is part of a general problem with all types of health care professionals—including nurses.

Some turnover is healthy in every institution. Too much stability can lead to stagnation and overall resistance to change. Innovation is an essential ingredient and the input of new nurses with new or at least different ideas can be a valuable asset. But there needs to be a balance; excessively high turnover does not permit innovations to take hold or changes to be implemented with enough follow-through to be significant.

The National Commission on Nursing (1981, p. 6) in its initial report lists four desired outcomes:

1. retaining nurses in practice
2. providing job satisfaction
3. maintaining and increasing the competence of nurses in practice
4. maintaining and improving the quality of nursing care.

This means that hospitals must look at both the internal and external causes of turnover. The internal causes include physicians' and administration's low acceptance of nurses, low pay and recognition, and unclear responsibilities. External causes can be summed up basically as a low career commitment on the part of many nurses, their high mobility today, and the problem of low supply and high demand.

This is a matter of more than just recruiting; it must be coupled with training and retraining those who are recruited. There also must be higher salaries and improvement in the nurses' overall environment.

"Training more nurses won't solve the problem until the underlying cause of the nursing shortage—high employee turnover—is solved. What is needed most is better pay and a hard-hitting marketing and public relations campaign aimed at physicians, not nurses, potential nursing students, or their high school counselors" (LaViolette, 1980).

In considering career ladders, significant major findings are reported by Price and Mueller (1981, p. 109). They state that nurses' opportunities to get ahead occupationally in hospitals decrease turnover. In their study, the determinants whose increase produced greater amounts of turnover include the facts that (a) many jobs are available outside of the hospital and (b) training prepares nurses to work in diverse occupational settings. Promotional opportunity was among the six determinants cited as important for at least three categories of nurses.

The results of another study on turnover (McCloskey, 1974) indicate that most nurse respondents want an opportunity to attend educational programs, continue course work for credit, seek career advancement, and have their work recognized by their peers and their supervisors. McCloskey suggests changing the traditional career advancement route that goes from staff nurse to team leader to head nurse and so on to a pattern related more closely to the levels of practice. This implies a clinical career ladder.

Overall there appears to be a significant relationship between nurses' turnover and career ladder programs. Nurses need and want room to grow in an organization.

APPLICATIONS OF CAREER LADDERS

Many applications of clinical ladders can be identified. Career ladders with clinical as well as other tracks are far less frequent. Huey (1982) provides a useful summary of the variety of programs being used. In a profile of seven career ladder programs around the nation, Huey compares key features of each, including salary differentials and promotion procedures. As Huey states, "In nursing, *clinical ladder* is fast becoming the most popular and broadly defined two-word phrase since *flexible hours* and *primary care*."

There is a clear distinction between a clinical ladder (single track) and a career ladder program (multitrack). Unfortunately, the distinction has become blurred because of the variety of combinations developed for individual situations.

The appendix includes a number of examples of ladder programs, some strictly clinical tracks, others multiple track. Of particular interest are the ways in which the job performance descriptions are developed to include the performance criteria that define the progressive steps (levels) on the clinical and other tracks and to serve the purposes of performance appraisal also. Nurse managers, administrators, and educators already have achieved great progress in these areas in the past decade with achievements of which their counterparts in other professions and industries might well be envious.

Another purpose of the appendix examples is to contrast the range of performance appraisal models being used—from highly sophisticated to deceptively simple. For example, contrast the appraisal forms presented in Appendixes G and I. There are valid reasons for both types, depending upon their intended purposes. From the standpoint of busy nurse managers, the simpler the better—if they serve the purpose. Many subscribe to the dictum, "The simplest things are often the most profound."

CRITERIA CHECKLISTS

Tables 6-1 and 6-2 are examples of tools the authors have developed to help in their evaluation and guidance of career ladder programs being planned or already in use.

For Discussion Purposes

The development and initiation of in-house or systemwide career ladders presents additional dilemmas for some nursing departments. These can relate to presumed obstacles to their use that may or may not exist. In any event, they should be addressed by the task force as a guide to an administrative decision regarding career ladders.

1. List the real and assumed roadblocks (identify which is which) to beginning a career ladder program.
2. Discuss how to remove such roadblocks.
3. Name the advantages and benefits of developing the career ladder program in conjunction with updating the performance appraisal program.
4. Cite any possible disadvantage.

Table 6-1 Criteria Checklist for Career Ladders

Items	Yes	No	Comments
1. Personnel policies, as relevant			
Labor contract provisions, if any			
2. Purpose, philosophy, and objectives			
3. Eligibility requirements (each level and category)			
4. Self-evaluation, based on performance description (forms).			
5. Manager evaluation, based on performance description (forms)			
6. Conference with nurse manager			
7. Application: forms and guidelines			
8. Weighting of recommendations for promotion			
9. Review process:			
a. Submit to Executive Council (or etc.) with recommendations			
b. Nurse manager recommendation			
c. Peer recommendations			
d. Criteria for accept/reject			
10. Number of available positions/unit			
11. Education and training required (core, specialty)			
12. Time required in present position (prepromotion)			
13. Credential weighting (i.e., recognition of B.S.N.)			
14. Experience weighting (prior job experience elsewhere)			
15. Consistency of career ladder policies with personnel and labor contract provisions regarding hiring, transfers, rehiring, promotion, etc.			
16. Other considerations:			

Table 6-2 Career Ladder Packet Considerations

Information and Forms	Yes	No	Comments
1. Instructions for use			
2. Job performance description			
3. Eligibility requirements			

Table 6-2 Career Ladder Packet Considerations (continued)

Information and Forms	Yes	No	Comments
4. Application form			
5. Evaluation forms (self, manager, peers)			
6. Recommendation form for action			
7. Record of education and training completed			
8. Skills checklist			
9. Process of notifying applicant of acceptance or rejection for ladder promotion			

Career Ladder Packet Processing

Identify:
1. Who will receive packet ....
2. Who will screen ....
3. Time frames ....
4. Review process ....

NOTES

Alexander, C.S.; Weisman, C.S.; & Chase, G.A. Determinants of staff nurses' perceptions of autonomy within different clinical contexts. *Nursing Research,* January/February 1982, *31*(1), 48–52.

Alt, J.; Bates, M.; Gilmore, M.A.; Houston, G.; & Stoner, R. New hope for "hands-on" nurses: Clinical promotions. *RN,* June 1980, *43*(6), 48–51.

Coogan, J. Nursing in the 90s: Autonomy and high morale . . . and about time, too. *Nursing 81,* November 1981, *11*(11), 22–24.

Ganong, J.M. More on clinical ladders. *Journal of Nursing Administration,* December 1982, *12*(12), 2.

Ganong, J.M. & Ganong, W.L. *HELP with wide-track careers in nursing.* Chapel Hill, N.C.: W.L. Ganong Co., 1977.

Ganong, J.M., & Ganong, W.L. *Nursing management* (2nd ed.). Rockville, Md.: Aspen Systems Corporation, 1980.

Ganong, J.M., & Ganong, W.L. *The G-GRAM: Newsletter for nurse managers and educators.* July/August 1982, *9*(4), 1. (a)

Ganong, J.M. & Ganong, W.L. *HELP with career ladders in nursing: Applying the wide-track careers concept.* Chapel Hill, N.C.: W.L. Ganong Co., 1982. (b)

Gulack, R. The main chance. *RN,* March 1983, *46*(3), 35–41.

Huey, F. Looking at ladders. *American Journal of Nursing,* 1982, *82*(10), 1520–1526.

Jaques, E. Taking time seriously in evaluating jobs. *Harvard Business Review,* September/October 1979, *57*(5), 124–132.

Knox, S. A clinical advancement program. *Journal of Nursing Administration,* July 1980, *10*(7), 29–33.

LaViolette, S. Multiunits boost nursing's clout. *Modern Healthcare,* January 1980, *10*(1), 50.

Lysaught, J.P. *An abstract for action.* New York: McGraw-Hill Book Company, 1970.

Lysaught, J.P. *Action in nursing: Progress in professional purpose.* New York: McGraw-Hill Book Company, 1973.

Lysaught, J.P. *Action in affirmation: Toward an unambiguous profession of nursing.* New York: McGraw-Hill Book Company, 1981.

McCloskey, J. Influence of rewards and incentives on staff nurse turnover. *Nursing Research,* May–June 1974, *23*(3).

National Commission on Nursing. *Initial report and preliminary recommendations.* Chicago: The Hospital Research and Educational Trust, 1981.

Price, J., & Mueller, C. *Professional turnover: The case for nurses.* Jamaica, N.Y.: Spectrum Publications, Inc., 1981.

Steck, A. The nursing shortage: An optimistic view. *Nursing Outlook,* May 1981, *29*(5), 302–304.

Wolf, G. Nursing turnover: Some causes and solutions. *Nursing Outlook,* April 1981, *29*(4), 233–236.

Zimmer, M. Rationale for a ladder for clinical advancement in nursing practice. *Journal of Nursing Administration,* November–December 1972, *11*(6), 19.

Chapter 7

Performance Appraisal of Students of Nursing

INTRODUCTION TO THE 'ESCAPE' MODEL

The Results-Oriented Performance Evaluation Program (ROPEP) model can be adapted for use in assessing the clinical performance of students of nursing, as discussed in this chapter. This has special significance for both faculty members and nurse managers, all of whom have urgent reasons to help assure the competency (productive effectiveness) of graduate nurses.

Student nurses must learn to do many things and do them at an acceptable level of competence. Satisfactory performance of any required activity, procedure, or process (including the nursing process itself) requires both knowledge and skill. The requisite knowledge and skills are taught by faculty members and clinical instructors who have the responsibility of helping the students to learn what they need to know and to do in order to pass each course and to graduate from the particular nursing program. While all students are accountable for their own learning, faculty members judge whether they pass or fail, graduate or do not graduate.

The model presented here is designed to assist students of nursing, faculty members, and nurse managers to evaluate the clinical performance of both student nurses and practicing nurses. The model is called Effective Student Clinical Achievement Performance Evaluation (ESCAPE). It provides a means to "Escape" from more conventional and sometimes unsatisfactory student appraisal methods. At the very least, it provides a useful supplement to existing techniques.

It focuses on clinical achievement—the ability to perform satisfactorily the "doing" aspects of patient care. Licensure examinations test for the knowledge deemed necessary to become a registered nurse (R.N.) or a licensed practical (vocational) nurse (L.P.N.). These examinations do not evaluate the basic skills necessary for satisfactory performance as a nurse. This was true for the older State Board Test Pool Examination (SBTPE) that was introduced in the mid-40s and used with revisions until the spring of 1982. The same thing is true also for the National Council Licensure Examination (NCLEX-RN and NCLEX-LPN), first used in the summer of 1982 (McCarty, 1982).

It has been the inadequate skill levels among nursing graduates (from whatever length of program) that have been disheartening to doctors, patients, and to nurse managers. There would seem to be no excuse for graduating and licensing nurses who cannot function at a minimal acceptable competency level. A systematic approach can be used to assure the highest competency level possible within the framework, resources, and strictures of each nursing program.

How ESCAPE Can Help

ESCAPE provides a means for:

- faculty members to establish clinical performance criteria and to evaluate the students' skill in performance as satisfactory or not satisfactory
- students to judge their own achievement in learning clinical performance skills
- employers to screen nursing applicants for their skill competencies in advance of being hired
- health care agencies to establish meaningful performance criteria for nurses to advance along the clinical track in a career ladder program
- staff development and inservice education departments to provide more meaningful skill development opportunities for nursing personnel in response to identified needs (as in connection with career ladder programs and quality assurance outcomes)
- nursing departments to reach a state of readiness that permits consideration of primary nursing as a viable alternative to other modes of care
- greater job satisfaction and motivation-through-the-work-itself as nursing personnel become real professionals at whatever job level.

The ESCAPE model can help nurse educators, students, inservice and continuing education faculty members, preceptors, nurse managers, and practitioners to modify present practices in the evaluation of clinical performance skills through:

- establishing specific, mutually understood, written, major performance expectations for use in clinical learning
- developing mutually agreed-upon statements of when student clinical performance is satisfactory in qualitative and quantitative terms
- participating effectively as facilitators in performance evaluation sessions with students
- using the self-evaluation approach effectively for self and others
- providing student counseling that builds upon each individual's assets
- relating learning contracts to effective student clinical achievement performance evaluation.

Views of Teaching and Learning

Rogers (1969) suggests that teachers should be careful not to interrupt a student who is learning just so they can do some teaching. This cautionary advice suggests a way of viewing the learning process that has profound implications for teaching students of nursing. The educator's view of teaching and learning necessarily is a major influence on the methods used to evaluate student achievements. Hence this is where to begin—with the teachers.

Figure 7-1 presents two contrasting ways of looking at the teacher-student relationship. The Teacher/Student diagram on the left is identified as Model T; the Facilitator/Learner diagram on the right is Model U. The letters *T* and *U* are used for several reasons. Visually, the two diagrams can be seen as a T and a U (on its side). T stands for Teacher, the more Traditional version. And while the Model T Ford was a great automobile and served its users well in its day, it has long since gone out of style. The U represents the full impact of YOU that goes into the learning-facilitator role in confluent education.

There is a similarity between these two role models and the role comparisons for managers as described by Myers, (1981). He identifies the authority-oriented manager as the one who plans, leads, and controls while the employee carries out the doing function. The goal-oriented manager, in contrast, permits employees the maximum amount of planning and controlling in connection with their doing while the manager serves as leader-facilitator.

The roles of teachers and of managers (in business, health care, government, and other institutions) have many common characteristics. Both groups, for example, are responsible for:

- overseeing the persons (students, employees) they supervise
- setting standards and goals

Figure 7-1 Roles of Teacher/Student and Facilitator/Learner

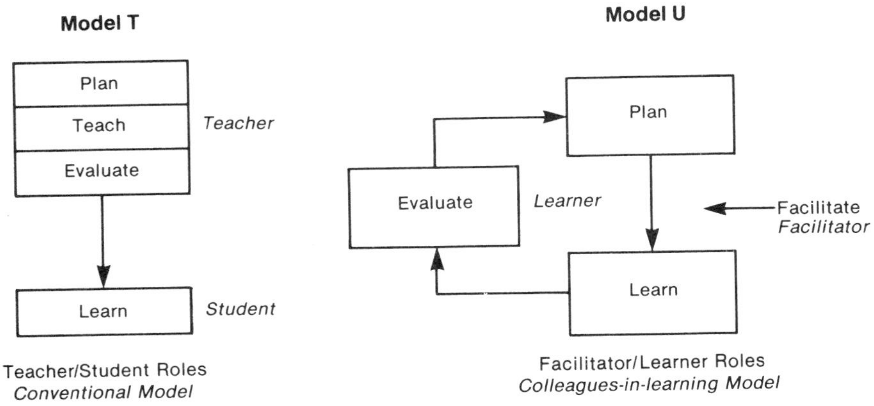

Model T

Model U

Plan

Teach   *Teacher*

Evaluate

Learn   *Student*

Plan

Evaluate   *Learner*

Learn

Facilitate
Facilitator

Teacher/Student Roles
Conventional Model

Facilitator/Learner Roles
Colleagues-in-learning Model

* Facilitating is used wherever necessary in Model U. It may be needed in planning, learning, or evaluating.

Source: Reprinted from *HELP with Effective Student Clinical Achievement Performance Evaluation* by Joan M. Ganong and Warren L. Ganong with permission of W.L. Ganong Co., © 1977, p. 6.

- assigning work to be done or learned
- providing suitable supplies, tools, and working or learning environment
- giving instructions
- maintaining discipline
- utilizing resources (time, money, facilities) effectively
- carrying out organizational policies
- solving problems and conflicts
- evaluating the performance of the students and employees
- recommending advancement as deserved.

In addition to these similarities, the range of leadership styles available is the same, as in the continuum of Figure 7-2. More specifically, Exhibit 7-1 lists some of the things a nurse manager/educator does, presented in two-column format for comparison of the nuances between the two leadership styles.

The teacher/manager analogy should be carried one step further. Among the ranks of managers, the real professionals are identified as those who are skilled developers of people—good teachers. Their people grow. Their

Figure 7-2 Range of Leadership Styles

Every leader has an individual style. This is as it should be. Every leader is an individual with personal attributes and assets to build upon. Successful nurse managers also recognize that thay can become skilled in several leadership styles. They learn to be flexible and to adapt their own style to meet the needs of different situations, individuals and groups. The diagram shows how leadership styles can range all the way from *telling* to *facilitating*.

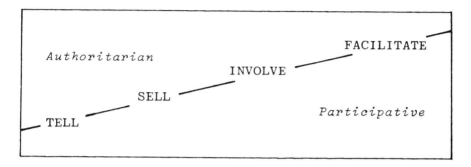

There are two main kinds of leadership: *authoritarian* and *participative. Authoritarian* leaders usually make their own decisions and *tell* employees what to do and how to do it. They seek obedience.

Participative leaders usually *involve* employees in problem-solving and decision-making whenever possible. They seek self direction and responsibility from employees. They make themselves available for help, materials, and information—for whatever employees need for patient care.

> A leader is best
> When people barely know that he exists
> Not so good when people obey and acclaim him
> Worst when they despise him
> *Fail to honour people*
> *They fail to honour you*
> But of a good leader, who talks little
> When his work is done, his aim fulfilled,
> They will all say: *We did this ourselves.*
> —Lao Tse, 600 BC

Source: Reprinted from *HELP with Managerial Leadership in Nursing: 101 Tremendous Trifles* (3rd ed.) by Joan M. Ganong and Warren L. Ganong with permission of W.L. Ganong Co., © 1980.

Exhibit 7-1 Role of the Nurse Manager/Nurse Educator

Authority-Oriented	*Goal-Oriented*
Set goals for subordinates, define standards and results expected.	Participate with people in problem solving and goal setting.
Give them information necessary to do their jobs.	Give them access to information they want.
Train them to do the job.	Create situations for optimum learning.
Explain rules and apply discipline to ensure conformity; suppress conflict.	Explain rules and consequences of violations; mediate conflict.
Stimulate subordinates through persuasive leadership.	Allow people to set challenging goals.
Develop and install new methods.	Teach methods improvement techniques to job incumbents.
Develop and free them for promotion.	Enable them to pursue and move into growth opportunities.
Reward achievements and punish failures.	Recognize achievements and help them learn from failures.

Source: Reprinted from *HELP with Effective Student Clinical Achievement Performance Evaluation* by Joan M. Ganong and Warren L. Ganong with permission of W.L. Ganong Co., © 1977, p. 9. (Adapted from Myers, 1970.)

people learn. Their people move up to broader management responsibilities because the managers have facilitated their growth, have helped them learn.

In a similar vein, the best teachers are likely to be those who are good managers. They make sure that adequate tools, supplies, and facilities are available for use by the students of whatever age or kind. They allow the learners to set goals. They give access to information the learners want. They aid self-evaluation. They recognize achievement. They help the students build on failures. They view themselves as facilitators of the learning process, as colleagues in learning. The ESCAPE method builds on these precepts.

ESCAPE Defined

ESCAPE is a performance evaluation method to measure the results of students' clinical experience and achievement compared with previously agreed-upon expectations and standards. Its key words are defined as follows:

Measure: determination of the degree of conformity with criteria of quality and quantity.
Results: consequences, outcomes.
Clinical: direct observation and treatment of patients.
Achievement: attained with effort.
Compared with: examined to note similarities and differences.
Agreed upon: developed jointly in advance with accord by teacher and student.
Expectations: specific clinical performance requirements (learning segments).
Standards: acknowledged measures of comparison for qualitative or quantitative value; criteria; norms.

Figure 7-3 demonstrates the operational model for ESCAPE. The diagram indicates how the student performance expectations and standards are developed out of the interaction of the value systems (personal and professional) of both teacher and learner. Similarly, it is the evaluation of clinical performance by both student and teacher that provides the basis for the performance evaluation conferences. The conferences lead to a joint resetting of objectives and a recycling of the process toward the ultimate goal of satisfactory performance.

ESCAPE provides a professionally satisfying alternative to more conventional or out-of-date clinical evaluation plans. Exhibit 7-2 is a comparison of the main characteristics of the older methods contrasted with the results-oriented focus of ESCAPE-type methods.

Implementing ESCAPE

Introducing ESCAPE in a school of nursing can be achieved in an orderly, step-by-step manner. Figure 7-4 provides a program performance plan and work sheet that identifies four implementation phases (see also Chapters 4 and 5 on ROPEP) as follows:

Phase I: The Initial Development
Phase II: Introduction

Figure 7-3 Operational Model for ESCAPE

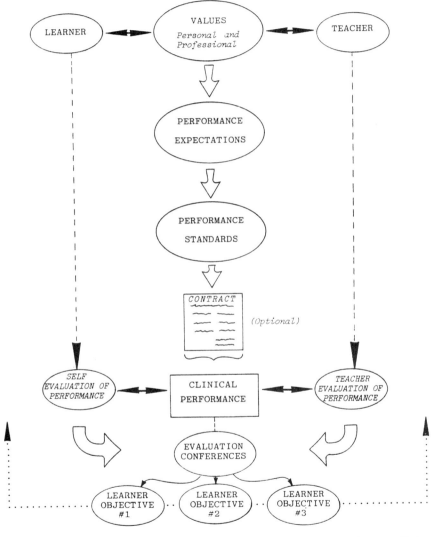

Source: Reprinted from *HELP with Effective Student Clinical Achievement Performance Evaluation* by Joan M. Ganong and Warren L. Ganong with permission of W.L. Ganong Co., © 1977, p. 15.

Exhibit 7-2 Comparison of Evaluation Methods

Conventional Method	Results-Oriented Method
Focus on:	*Focus on:*
● Personality traits	● Specific performance criteria and objectives
● Weaknesses	● Strengths (limited criticism)
● One-way evaluation	● Two-way evaluation
● Periodic evaluation	● Day-to-day coaching with periodic evaluation
● Looking back	● Looking back + forward to future

Phase III: The First Evaluation Cycle
Phase IV: The Continuing Evaluation Cycle

INITIAL DEVELOPMENT: PHASE I

When faculty members feel that the time has come to review and revise their student clinical performance evaluation process, one of the first steps is to form either a task force, a committee, or a project team. This group should consist of faculty members and selected student representatives. Once it has determined its goals and objectives, it can clarify the needs identified for an ESCAPE approach.

While these needs will vary from one college or school of nursing to another, the broad reasons for undertaking an ESCAPE program include the following:

- The present performance evaluation system is not meeting expectations of faculty and/or students.
- Complaints by faculty or students are significant enough in number to warrant review and revision of the program.
- The existing evaluation system does not meet standards and criteria of the National League for Nursing.
- The existing performance evaluation system relies too heavily on a complicated rating system.
- The existing system relies more heavily on personality traits than on behavioral criteria.
- Specific objectives citing requested or required behavioral changes in clinical performance are not identified in the existing process.

The working group also should consider spending time identifying the values of its task force members, especially in reference to performance

Figure 7-4 ESCAPE: Program Performance Plan and Worksheet

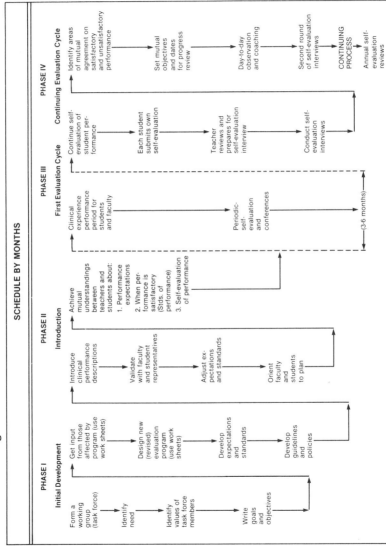

Source: Reprinted from *HELP with Effective Student Clinical Achievement Performance Evaluation* by Joan M. Ganong and Warren L. Ganong with permission of W.L. Ganong Co., © 1977, p. 79.

evaluation or appraisal. As indicated in the operational model for ESCAPE (Figure 7-3, supra), the personal and professional values of faculty and students play an important role in determining the entire performance evaluation process.

Values can be seen as determinants of all kinds of conduct that could be called social behavior. That includes, among other things, attitudes, evaluations, moral judgments, justification of self and others, and the comparison of self with others. Values are guides and determinants of social attitudes and ideologies on the one hand and of social behavior on the other. They guide and determine action, attitudes toward objects and situations, evaluations, judgments, and justifications, as well as comparisons and attempts to influence others (Rokeach, 1973, pp. 24–25).

Values, as guides to behavior, evolve and mature as the individuals do. Values are a part of living and operate in complex circumstances involving more than simple extremes of right and wrong, good or bad, true or false. Behavior is guided by values under conditions that typically involve conflicting demands; these conditions require weighing and balancing and, finally, action that reflects the multitude of forces at work. Values seldom function in a pure and abstract form. Complicated judgments are involved. What is really valued is reflected in the outcome of life as it is finally lived by the individual. Values can be based on three processes: choosing, prizing, and acting. Collectively, these define valuing. The results of the valuing process are called values (Raths, Harmin, and Simon, 1966, pp. 27–30).

Working group discussions concerning values should take into consideration such points as the purpose of evaluation and peoples' reaction to it, how people learn, acceptance vs. approval, the role of criticism in the achievement of goals, the role of the teacher in the learning process, individual differences among students and faculty, the relationship between performance and knowledge, and the role of self-evaluation vs. evaluations done only by the faculty.

The written goals and objectives of the ESCAPE program can be finalized following the identification of values. The goals should state the overall purpose or aim of the program. Both goals and objectives should take into account the fact that ESCAPE can provide a means to:

- establish clinical performance criteria and evaluation of the students' skills as satisfactory or not satisfactory
- enable students to judge their own achievement and learning of clinical performance skills through self-evaluation
- utilize criteria-based statements of major performance expectations for use in any clinical learning setting

- allow for results-oriented faculty-student performance evaluation sessions
- provide student counseling concerning clinical performance that builds on each student's assets
- offer the option of learning contracts
- utilize mutually agreed-upon objectives for the behavior changes identified as necessary to meet the criteria established for performance.

The goals and objectives of the ESCAPE program should go hand in hand with those of the working group. Once the program is established, the group disbands with, it hopes, its targets met. The goals and objectives of the program, however, are continuing and will remain in place as amended until another revision is necessary.

The preparation of the clinical performance expectations, involving both the use and analysis of the work sheets and the development of expectations and standards, is the longest part of Phase I of ESCAPE.

Student Clinical Performance Expectations

A Student Clinical Performance Expectation is a statement of the major expectations (grouped by persons for whom they are carried out), with measurable standards of satisfactory performance. The student clinical performance expectation is similar to a job performance description for a practicing registered nurse. In its final form the Student Clinical Performance Expectation is intended to describe the responsibilities and expectations (behavioral objectives), with identified measures (criteria) of satisfactory performance of a student who expects to pass the clinical part of a nursing course. It is best prepared by a process of performance analysis carried out by selected faculty members, with student input. Its purpose is to produce student-faculty agreement and understanding regarding the clinical performance expected of the students to make possible meaningful continuing evaluation of performance.

The emphasis in preparing the expectations is in reaching a mutual understanding as to who is to do what for whom how well so that later there can be an agreement on what was learned and demonstrated in actual clinical performance. One benefit of such a document is the preparation and involvement process itself. The paperwork (the final form) is important because it facilitates mutual understanding but the involvement process is critical if the form is to be a meaningful part of the evaluation/learning program.

Exhibit 7-3 is a "Performance Expectations Work Sheet." It is an adjunct to the clinical course behavioral objectives and can be helpful in

Exhibit 7-3 Performance Expectations Work Sheet

EFFECTIVE
STUDENT
CLINICAL
ACHIEVEMENT
PERFORMANCE
EVALUATION

Expectations *Major Performance Expectations*	*Criteria* *Performance Is Satisfactory When:*
1.	1.
2.	2.
3.	3.
4.	4.
5.	5.

Source: Reprinted from *HELP with Performance Appraisal: A Results-Oriented Approach* by Joan M. Ganong and Warren L. Ganong with permission of W.L. Ganong Co., © 1975, p. 20.

accumulating and agreeing upon clinical expectations and standards. This form can be completed by any students who have had clinical learning experiences in the nursing education program. It is recommended that if possible three parties be involved in using these work sheets during the initial development cycle—teachers, students, and nurses from a clinical practice setting. The practicing R.N. from the clinical facility who could contribute the most probably would be a recent graduate who has had time to sharpen clinical skills on the job and whose memory still is fresh with the details of what it was essential to acquire to reach a "satisfactory" level of performance.

Exhibit 7-4 is an example of major performance expectations for a second-level student, together with appropriate behavioral criteria for satisfactory work.

Exhibit 7-4 Performance Expectations Work Sheet

(Example for Level II Student)

Major Performance Expectations	Performance Is Satisfactory (Criteria) When:
To Patient	
1. Uses assessment skills and tools to determine problems, needs of assigned patients.	1. Some patient needs and problems are identified correctly as direct result of interviewing, observing, and caring for patient. Findings are corroborated by clinical instructor.
2. Formulates a plan of care for patient's identified needs and problems. Uses planning skills and tools.	2. Care plan is discussed and documented for each assigned patient. Care is based on assessment. Plan is corroborated by clinical instructor.
3. Uses a problem-oriented approach to patient care.	3. Patient care and chart reflect the problem-solving steps used in identifying problems. Goals and objectives are set with patient. Problems and solutions are documented correctly.
4. Implements a plan of care.	4. Care plan is followed for assigned patients. Results of plan are seen in the patient and on the progress notes and flow sheets.
5. Evaluates the care that the patient has received.	5. Changes in patient as result of planned care are identified correctly. Plan is adjusted according to new findings.

Source: The authors are indebted to Carol H. Phillips, R.N., M.P.H., for preparing this example while an instructor in the Watts Hospital School of Nursing in Durham, N.C.

The Learning Contract and ESCAPE

The use of the learning contract is optional in ESCAPE. As shown in the "Operational Model for ESCAPE" (Figure 7-3 supra), the contract can be a natural step in following through with the performance expectations and standards that have been agreed upon. (Table 7-1 is an example of a learning contract work sheet.)

A contract has been defined as:

> [a] business-like arrangement whereby the instructor defines the performance required for each grade, the student identifies the performance level to which he will work, and signs a contract in which the instructor is committed to awarding the predetermined grade if the student attains the appropriate performance level (Harvey, 1972).

According to Combs, Avila, and Purkey (1971, p. 117) responsibility is learned from being given responsibilities. Contracting can help students learn to take responsibility for their own behavior.

While there are several approaches to contracting, some teachers have difficulty in accommodating themselves to the concept. Those who use contracting have to be willing to let students experiment with the idea themselves, possibly making mistakes in the contracting process. A student who contracts for a C but does B work will learn to set higher sights next time. Another student who contracts for an A and does only C work has not fulfilled the contract and may learn to set sights more realistically next time.

Both teacher and student have a responsibility to respect the terms of the contract and to allow the process to be a useful learning experience. In the final analysis the student must have earned the grade, based upon the terms of the contract, not just received a grade given by the teacher. A failing grade should mean that the student has failed to fulfill the contract, not that the teacher has failed the student. Some failures are inevitable in almost any course. A failure is not a disgrace. Most persons, with suitable guidance, are able to learn through their failure experiences. Students need to know it is OK to fail once in a while. If a learning contract is used well, it facilitates success for the student in a businesslike way.

Suggestions for Contracting

Teachers who want to initiate contracting with students should:

- avoid identifying only quantity in the contract performance requirements; identify quality requirements, too

Table 7-1 Clinical Learning Contract Work Sheet

Contract Arrangements: The contract is a mutual agreement whereby the teacher defines the course purpose, objectives, and the clinical performance required for each grade; the learner identifies own objectives and the level to which he or she will work. Both agree on the conditions and sign the contract. The teacher is committed to awarding the predetermined grade if the learner attains the appropriate performance level, thus fulfilling the requirements of the contract. Failure to meet the contract provisions nullifies the contract.

COURSE OBJECTIVES: Upon completion the student will be able to: For Nursing III:	A	CRITERIA FOR GRADE PERFORMANCE B	C
1. Utilize the components of the nursing process in giving care to patients during clinical practice.	Assess and plan patient data and document on 8-hour basis according to concept. State the concept and interpret it correctly. Utilize evaluation component of nursing process. Tie in with actual teaching of patient. Adjust care plan as necessary.	Assess and plan patient data and document for 24-hour period on patient records on 8-hour basis. State the concept correctly. Utilize evaluation component of nursing process. Make some adjustments in plan.	Assess and plan patient data for 24-hour period and document on a daily basis. Make adjustments in plan with help.
2. Communicate effectively with nursing staff regarding assigned patients.	Use written, oral, and listening skills effectively in patient report and conference.	Use some written, oral, and listening skills in report and conference.	Make at least limited use of written, oral, and listening skills.
3. Interpret and utilize theory of the nursing process.	Demonstrate skilled use of entire nursing process repeatedly with all assigned patients.	Demonstrate use of entire nursing process with most assigned patients.	Demonstrate use of some of the nursing process on some assigned patients and partially on others.

SIGNED BY (STUDENT): _____ DATE _____ (TEACHER): _____ DATE _____

Source: Reprinted with permission from *HELP with Effective Student Clinical Achievement Performance Evaluation* by Joan M. Ganong and Warren L. Ganong with permission of W.L. Ganong Co., © 1977, p. 66.

Performance Appraisal of Students of Nursing 157

- require that, once the grade is set, the student fulfill the agreed-upon terms or the contract is broken
- combine classroom and clinical performance requirements
- give students the option to contract or not to contract
- require evidence for each performance item; this must be discussed, clarified, and agreed upon so that the student knows whether the teacher will observe or document the performance.

Possible Outcomes of Contracting

There are numerous results possible through the contracting process, among them those that produce:

- increased involvement by the student in decisions and planning
- increased student satisfaction
- increased creative efforts by student
- increased responsibility for student
- decreased competition with other students
- maximized potential of the student

Singer (1972) provides the following overview and advantages of learning contracts:

Learning Contracts: Viable Alternative

The most useful current work on the subject of grade reform is *Wad Ja Get?* (H. Kirschenbaum et al, Hart, 1971), which outlines a number of alternatives to current grading practices. The particular grading system which is most ideal or most feasible will, of course, vary from place to place. However, in my experience the contract grading system is the most widely applicable and optimal alternative.

The basic idea is that the instructor and student contract with each other for specified accomplishments for specified grades. The grades may be A, B, P, 4, or whatever. The student is not evaluated relative to others, but merits a given grade by reaching an absolute level of accomplishment. The contract may vary from being completely instructor determined, which would amount to unitized instruction, to being wholly student determined, which would amount to students' deciding their own goals and assigning themselves marks.

In a college class, for instance, a contract might consist of attending class, reading and reporting on two texts, and doing an adequate project or paper for an A, or a B if one item is not fulfilled. On an elementary level, Montessori or free school classrooms typically use a version of the contract approach in which the child and the teacher discuss what the child wants to do and what they think he can accomplish. The obligatory part of the contract in this case derives from the personal relationship between the child and the teachers.

The contract grading system has the following advantages:

1. The instructor and the student have a wide latitude within which to work out their own balance of structure and freedom.
2. Since students can achieve high grades by working to achieve specified concrete goals, they are more motivated toward their achievement.
3. Creativity and substantive accomplishment are encouraged by this system. It is a human condition that self-determination is more motivating than behavior enforced by others.
4. Competitiveness, comparative evaluations, and time pressure are alleviated.
5. Under the contract system, grades may even be legitimate measuring devices. There is at least a prima facie rationale for their representing substantive achievement and measuring a student's motivation.
6. Under this system students usually get high grades and do not have to fear low grades. School becomes more rewarding.
7. The contract system is easy to defend against administrative questioning. There are usually no rules against it. It is becoming widespread in one form or another and thus is legitimized through usage, like everything else in education.

You can present administrators with clear rationales for using this system and present for their examination piles of contracts students have written and work they have produced. In my experience administrative hassle stops at this point. (Singer, 1972).

In summary, a contract is an enforceable agreement—a covenant. The use of learning contracts between student and teacher is a method of assuring student involvement in goal setting. At the beginning of a course, teachers contract with students for the grade each one will receive. The contract may specify what books will be read, what types of assignments (including clinical) will be completed, what methods of examination will be used, and so on. The teacher agrees to give the contract grade, whether A, B, or C, when the student presents evidence or certification of having carried out the contract terms.

". . . when students perceive that they are free to follow their own goals, most of them invest more of themselves in their effort, work harder, and retain and use more of what they have learned. . . ." (Rogers, 1969).

INTRODUCTION: PHASE II

Once the performance expectations, standards, and criteria have been developed, they are introduced and validated with faculty and student representatives. At that point the important thing is to get as much feedback as possible so that, if necessary, additional drafts of the clinical performance descriptions can be written.

It is the function of the working group members to act as ESCAPE ambassadors at this point. That is to say, they should hold as many group sessions as are necessary to make certain that the wording in the document is clear and understood by all. This kind of involvement is invaluable to the success of the program later on. It is wise for group members to listen to and accept all kinds of positive and negative feedback that can be taken back to their discussions and used for any revisions that may be necessary.

While this beginning part of Phase II may be time consuming, it is being implemented with the understanding that once the program is in effect, it will be there to stay a while—perhaps over a number of years, with minor revisions as necessary. This makes the efforts of the group much more rewarding and gives the program a better chance to be evaluated thoroughly later. The time spent in adjusting the expectations and standards thus is worthwhile in terms of the involvement of faculty and students in the preparation process, as well as in the final product itself.

Once all the final adjustments are made, both faculty and students need to be separately and collectively oriented to the ESCAPE program. The orientation includes the philosophy, goals, and objectives of the program; the program plan; guidelines; policies; forms; and time frames.

Exhibit 7-5 is a "Teacher's Guide and Checklist" for use in conducting a self-evaluation with a student on performance expectations in role clarification and performance evaluation. This form is given to faculty members and students so both groups have a clear understanding of the flow of the ESCAPE program. It is necessary first to reach an understanding

Exhibit 7-5 Teacher's Guide & Checklist for Use in Student Self-
Evaluation Session

A. Student and teacher reach understanding regarding each of the performance expectations and standards. The teacher:
_____1. Reviews performance expectations and standards.
_____2. Asks for comments and questions.
_____3. Clarifies and amplifies the performance expectations.
_____4. Explains the self-evaluation procedure and form.
B. Teacher provides for self-evaluation:
_____1. Gives student a copy of the self-evaluation forms.
_____2. Sets a date for completion. (Teacher also completes one.)
_____3. Obtains from student the self-evaluation form with written comments regarding how well student thinks each performance expectation has been met.
C. Teacher conducts self-evaluation conference:
_____1. Sets a date for the discussion conference.
_____2. Meets with student and *listens* to all comments.
_____3. Agrees whenever possible with student's own evaluation of performance. Compliments as appropriate.
_____4. Disagrees as necessary, each time asking for explanation of student's comments. Indicates why teacher feels performance was better than, or not as good as, student's own evaluation.
_____5. Reaches agreement on performance expectations that need strengthening.
_____6. Listens to student's suggestion for own improvement. Provides suggestions and help for improvement.
_____7. Discusses suggestions for specific follow-through action.
_____8. Reaches mutual agreement with student on objectives.

Source: Adapted from *HELP with Effective Student Clinical Achievement Performance Evaluation* by Joan M. Ganong and Warren L. Ganong with permission of W.L. Ganong Co., © 1977, p. 15.

---

between students and teachers on each of the performance expectations and standards.

Review of Performance Expectations and Standards

This step can be carried out with students either individually or as a group, depending on the size of the class. In any event, it will be simplified if the students already have assisted in the preparation of the statements that are used in the performance expectations. Even for those who have participated, at this time the teachers will have to review the performance expectations with each and every student and to continue this as a part of every periodic evaluation discussion.

Where there is lack of clarity about what is expected and what the behavioral criteria require, there is room for student misunderstanding. Since this must be avoided at all costs, the review is an important step.

Solicitation of Comments and Questions

This step seeks to encourage open exploration of what the student's clinical experience is all about. It should include what has to be done for whom and how well. How teachers handle this kind of discussion depends greatly on their individual style and communication skills. What works well for one individual may not do so for another.

An influential factor in the level of communication is the attitude teachers bring to the discussion. That is why so much time is spent here on the importance of values. Instructors' attitude and values will be apparent in their behavior during the discussions. It is, after all, the teachers who must set the climate for open discussion. It should be kept in mind that the important element is clarity and mutual understanding of what is expected of the student in a clinical setting.

Clarification and Amplification

This step essentially builds on what the teachers have been doing already in the review of the performance expectations. It is essential for the first time that the students know for certain that this program now is real. It becomes a part of their total learning experience. So this step should not be hurried. Whatever time it takes will be well spent.

In the interest of clarity, the teacher at this stage should be asking repeatedly, "What does this mean to you?" At the same time the teacher should be seeking understanding from the student by asking, "Tell me in your own words what this means." It also may be necessary to keep reiterating, "The reason we are doing this is so that both you and I have the same understanding about your clinical experience and what we can expect of each other."

Specific examples can be both colorful and descriptive, so it helps to use as many of them as possible from the teacher's own experience. Once again, the point of this step is to achieve clarity of understanding.

The Procedure Explained

The self-evaluation aspect of ESCAPE is a theme that requires emphasis throughout every step of the process. For example, the teacher comments to the student:

> The reason for our having this kind of a self-evaluation program
> is so that you can feel comfortable during your clinical experi-
> ences without having me looking over your shoulder all the time.

Most people don't like the idea of a clinical instructor being a "snoopervisor." I don't like it either. The best way for both of us to get along together is for us to understand what both of us (you and me) consider to be satisfactory performance of your expectations. So let's take a look at these again.

The teacher then explains that:

- The first regular clinical performance evaluation discussion will include all of the performance expectations.
- Subsequent regular evaluations will focus on the performance results that are exceptional (good) because they are outstanding or (poor) because they do not meet the standard of satisfactory performance. This is the exception principle. All other performance results require no attention because they all are satisfactory.
- Clinical performance evaluation really is a continuing day-to-day process. Thus there are likely to be many occasions when the performance expectations will be used to clarify questions, to remind each other of performance standards, to help plan learning experiences for skill improvement, and for other learning-related purposes. This is especially timely during preclinical and postclinical conferences.

The Self-Evaluation Forms

At this point the student should be given a copy of the self-evaluation forms. An example is provided in Exhibit 7-6, titled, "Quarterly Student Clinical Evaluation." It should be explained that these forms are filled out individually by the student and the faculty member. In some cases students may wish to turn these in before the evaluation or appraisal conference date. In other instances, for reasons of their own, they may choose to simply bring the self-evaluation form with them to the conference. So much here depends on the level of trust between the student and teacher. Nevertheless, it should be clear that the forms based on the agreed-upon expectations and standards and criteria will form the basis for the conference.

Completion Date for First Self-Evaluation

Dates for clinical evaluation conferences may have been established already in the school or college of nursing. The ESCAPE program is intended to fit in with those dates.

Exhibit 7-6 Quarterly Student Clinical Evaluation

NAME _____ DATES from _____ to _____

CLINICAL ROTATION AREA _____ COURSE _____

A SATISFACTORY level of clinical performance must be maintained in order to pass this course. Students may make errors in the process of learning. A pattern of errors, however, will be considered UNSATISFACTORY.

INSTRUCTIONS: Check the appropriate level of performance for each objective and write in space provided behaviors indicative of the level checked.

The student:

1. Transfers and applies knowledge to care of patients.
   ___Satisfactory   ___Unsatisfactory
   Behaviors:

2. Makes careful and accurate observations of patient and environment.
   ___Satisfactory   ___Unsatisfactory
   Behaviors:

3. Adapts readily to each nursing care situation.
   ___Satisfactory   ___Unsatisfactory
   Behaviors:

4. Relates therapeutically to patients.
   ___Satisfactory   ___Unsatisfactory
   Behaviors:

5. Relates well to others on health care team.
   ___Satisfactory   ___Unsatisfactory
   Behaviors:

6. Shows a developing sense of responsibility for nursing functions within limit of own knowledge and experience.
   ___Satisfactory   ___Unsatisfactory
   Behaviors:

Exhibit 7-6 continued

7. Demonstrates responsibility for own clinical learning by:
   a) Attendance for clinical experience.
   ___Satisfactory   ___Unsatisfactory
   Behaviors:

   b) Punctuality for clinical experience.
   ___Satisfactory   ___Unsatisfactory
   Behaviors:

   c) Preparation for clinical nursing assignment, including nursing care planning.
   ___Satisfactory   ___Unsatisfactory
   Behaviors:

   d) Seeks new learning experiences.
   ___Satisfactory   ___Unsatisfactory
   Behaviors:

8. Gives safe, accurate care to patients.
   ___Satisfactory   ___Unsatisfactory
   Behaviors:

9. Organizes delivery of nursing care in a logical sequence based on the needs of patients within allotted time.
   ___Satisfactory   ___Unsatisfactory
   Behaviors:

10. Sets priorities appropriately in giving care to patients.
    ___Satisfactory   ___Unsatisfactory
    Behaviors:

Exhibit 7-6 continued

11. Records and reports accurate, concise, descriptive, and factual information.
___Satisfactory   ___Unsatisfactory
Behaviors:

12. Additional Comments

Appearance:

Other:

Student's Signature _____ Date _____

Instructor's Signature _____ Date _____

Source: Reprinted from *HELP with Effective Student Clinical Achievement Performance Evaluation* by Joan M. Ganong and Warren L. Ganong with permission of W.L. Ganong Co., © 1977, pp. 75–78.

In any event, a date for completing the forms by both teacher and student must be set and understood by both parties. In some instances the date for completing the first self-evaluation may be set soon after this initial conference. Much depends on the readiness of the individual student. The clinical instructor will have to judge how soon to allow this step to be completed.

The Initial Self-Evaluation Session

As noted earlier, it may well be that the students prefer to bring the self-evaluation form with them so they may speak about them during the conference without the teachers' having seen them in advance. Depending on where the students are in the program, they should be reminded of the exception principle just mentioned. It will become increasingly important to focus on all aspects of the expectations, standards, and criteria during the first evaluation cycle.

The teacher should encourage students to discuss their efforts at self-evaluation if they want to do so. It may well be the first time that they have been faced with this situation and may feel uncertain as to what to do. It should be kept in mind that many students are not used to being asked how they feel about their own performance; rather, they are used to being told how they are performing from the perception of the teacher.

While the teacher's input is a necessary part of evaluation, all students want to know how they are doing from the teacher's point of view. However, it is necessary to reiterate that this program is an attempt to help build accountability for self in nursing students.

They may need nothing more than time with the teacher to explain how they think they are progressing. This may be done because they need encouragement or approval or even just kind words. Such an interchange before an actual evaluation discussion can be very valuable in preparing both students and teacher for a productive follow-through of the interview.

The steps discussed in this approach have included reaching an understanding between students and teacher regarding each of the performance expectations and standards and providing for self-evaluation. The last section of the Checklist is put to use later in Phases III and IV. Phase II concludes once the program has been completely introduced.

As the lead-in to Phase III, the students begin their actual clinical experience for whatever period of time has been established. This includes periodic self-evaluation and conferences that are less formal in nature. In most schools and colleges of nursing, sessions of this kind are going on as postconferences following each clinical experience. The necessity for day-to-day coaching, especially in terms of formative feedback to the student, cannot be overemphasized (Tosti, 1980). (See Chapter 1 for a detailed discussion of this.)

There should be no surprises in the conferences for either student or teacher. As the student is fulfilling the stated expectations, behavioral standards, and criteria, the teacher should be giving feedback on how that individual is coming along. Individual "conferences" that take only minutes and may be held while standing at the elevator, having a cup of coffee, or walking to and from the clinical setting can be invaluable as a part of the entire growth and evaluation process. This is especially true in programs where the student will have limited opportunity to repeat assigned learning experiences.

FIRST EVALUATION CYCLE: PHASE III

As discussed earlier, teachers introducing ESCAPE will find that each student is at a different stage of readiness based on the extent of their participation in Phase I and their contribution to the development of their performance expectations. Newer students, and others who for one reason or another were not able to participate directly in Phase I and/or Phase II will be far less informed and will require the greatest amount of initial orientation to the first use of the performance expectations for the self-evaluation procedure.

The emphasis in the ESCAPE method is on self-evaluation and accountability. "A real method of instilling the potential of accountability is to remove the crutch of inspection and instead directly identify the performance of the work with the individual" (Herzberg, 1974). To do less is to perpetuate the record of frustration that has been characteristic of traditional student appraisal and performance review plans in so many learning institutions, including schools of nursing. The student self-evaluation is accompanied by the faculty appraisal, assuring a two-way results-oriented evaluation.

ESCAPE is similar to the Nursing Audit in many respects. Both are evaluative processes. Both establish standards of performance for measurement purposes. Both seek to provide criteria that will lead to student performance results that assure the optimum learning and delivery of patient care services.

Experiences in developing and using performance measures provide excellent learning opportunities for teachers, clinical instructors, nurse practitioners, and students, regardless of any other outcomes. The standards and criteria produced from these initial efforts can be modified and improved as they are used for evaluation purposes. Even more useful than the standards themselves is the process of developing, using, and redefining them. The standards simply are the means toward the end of more effective learning and skill development.

CONDUCTING A SELF-EVALUATION CONFERENCE

The first conference using the ESCAPE method is an important one. Steps are outlined in the "Teacher's Guide and Checklist" (Exhibit 7-5, supra, Section C). That section contains eight steps, each of which is important in achieving either (1) assurance that the student's performance is indeed satisfactory and perhaps exemplary in every way, or (2) that the student is not meeting some of the expectations, standards, and criteria and there is room for improvement.

The Behavioral Objectives Approach

Teachers have been setting objectives and writing lesson plans from time immemorial. Students in their own ways have been thinking about objectives, too. When they have done so, and have had opportunities for comparison, the objectives of the students and the teachers sometimes have been in agreement, sometimes at variance.

Behavioral objectives are a special way of stating the goals of a particular teaching/learning process. They focus on the students and what they expect to get out of their learning experiences. Such objectives, therefore, state the type of behavior (outcome) expected of the students (by the teacher and/or the students) as a result of the teaching/learning process. Behavior is any activity, usually visible but not necessarily so, displayed or engaged in by a learner.

The implications of this are that the students, with such a personal stake in the teaching/learning process, need direct involvement in the setting of behavioral objectives and in measuring the success of their educational experiences from their own point of view.

Confluent Objectives for Confluent Behavior

A behavior is a behavior. A person acts holistically, as a whole person. Behavior is not seen as cognitively motivated on the one hand and affectively motivated on the other. The thrust of confluent education is to recognize and build upon the merged flowing together of thinking and feeling in life and work activities and in learning projects.

Learning objectives are viewed in the same behaviorally oriented context. Yes, it is true that behavior (and learning) are affected by a person's values, attitudes, beliefs, likes, and dislikes. Yes, it is true that learning (and behavior) are influenced by a person's knowledge and understanding. The task then is to build objectives that incorporate both of these influences. That does not mean nurse educators should get carried away and spend their energies devising esoteric statements of increasingly refined minutiae that contribute little to the learning process.

After all, a prime reason for having objectives prepared by, or in conjunction with, the students is to provide a means for both teachers and learners—especially the latter—to evaluate the success of the learning projects. Experience indicates that such an approach leads to more successful learning.

Objectives and Expectations

Expectations are particular kinds of behavioral learning objectives as related to the clinical skills required for a nursing education level. Objectives may be as limited as what is required for the satisfactory completion of a performance expectation. Or an objective may be one step in a series of steps that must be accomplished to attain a long-range or short-range goal.

Two examples of objectives:

1. The nursing student will give an intramuscular injection at the correct site and angle, with accurate dosage, aseptic technique, and minimum discomfort for the patient. (This is a performance expectation type of objective.)
2. The nurse educator will meet with students individually to review their self-evaluations as Step C of the ESCAPE procedure. (This is a program performance plan type of objective as part of attaining this year's goals with students.)

A useful "Objectives Work Sheet" is shown in Exhibit 5-2, supra. It can be used in connection with the planning and follow-through of both types of objectives—those related to (1) specific performance expectations and (2) longer range goals. One of these work sheets prepared for each objective serves as a planning and evaluative tool in connection with discussions between student and teacher. Each work sheet remains active for the life of the objective to which it pertains. It is revised as required or when target dates have to be extended.

When an objective is terminated for whatever reason (completed successfully, cancelled for some cause, phased out, or merged with another project), the related work sheet, properly annotated, becomes a historical student record for follow-through purposes. Each one represents a promise (good intentions) kept or unfulfilled. A collection of such sheets for any student (dated and signed) can become an important supplement to other critical incident and anecdotal records.

THE CONTINUING EVALUATION CYCLE: PHASE IV

The early phases of setting up and initiating ESCAPE are necessary for a successful clinical performance evaluation program. This is true for most teacher/manager programs. The preparation and beginning phases seem more time consuming than the use and maintenance of the program. Yet suitable help and guidance can minimize the time requirements for introducing the program and completing the performance expectations. An additional benefit of such help is the training of the teaching personnel who will coordinate the program and serve as organizational resource persons.

The ESCAPE/objectives relationship discussed earlier demonstrates how the clinical performance evaluation concept is broadened to include all aspects of student goals, the regular expectations as well as those periodically assigned. The latter are a natural outgrowth of the ESCAPE method since some objectives will relate to action needed to assure a satisfactory level of performance for one or more major performance expectations.

There is a danger, however, in emphasizing deficiencies. Certainly errors and grossly unsatisfactory performance cannot be allowed to continue. But the focus needs to be upon identifying and building upon the strengths of individuals. This is especially true for the student who is, after all, in the process of learning, and may make an occasional error while doing so.

This phase (see Figure 7-4, supra) considers the continuous evaluation process once the initial developmental stages of ESCAPE have been completed and the first self-evaluation cycle has occurred. An important reminder is that ESCAPE is not a once-a-semester enforced appraisal routine scheduled to coincide only with the completion of a course. It is instead a day-by-day teaching tool and learning aid to assist student progress in the clinical program.

A SUMMARY OF THE ESCAPE MODEL

Learning to Be Useful

The health care system needs nurses who have a desire to do something useful, productive, and respected. Students of nursing learn to use new knowledge, skills, and feelings in a wide variety of clinical settings within the system. As learners, they cry out for a climate that expects and recognizes top performance. Such a climate is one in which there is room for innovation, self-growth, questions and answers, and a sense of partnership and cooperation.

ESCAPE attempts to help students learn the value of self-evaluation of their performance in the clinical area where there are patients and other health care personnel. ESCAPE focuses on strengths to improve weaknesses and encourages goal setting and achievement by identifying performance expectations and standards of satisfactory performance. In effect, it encourages both students and faculty to feel useful, productive, and respected.

Clinical instructors help to create a top performance climate. The relationships they establish and maintain with nursing service personnel, and with students and patients, all contribute to this climate.

Satisfactory vs. Top Performance

Why does ESCAPE use measures of "satisfactory" performance standards instead of some higher goal of excellence? Perhaps the reasons already are evident:

- There is a need to be realistic in regard to what level of clinical performance should be expected.
- The "satisfactory" standard is a demanding one, especially when the measure is "no errors" in the critical tasks of patient care.
- Teachers and students have learned through experience the fallacies and hazards of more complicated evaluation methods.
- Excellence in performance often occurs in spite of, not because of, an evaluation program designed as a teacher control system. Excellence is achieved by students who take pride in their performance and who get satisfaction from what they do.

This last reason is highly significant. Certainly health care institutions and schools of nursing need to strive for top performance and excellence today more than ever before. Competition, always a motivational factor in any organization, is affecting hospitals and schools. Health care organizations need as many people as possible who will contribute to creating a climate for top clinical performance results by students who become the nurses of the future. This is the road to true productivity in nursing practice.

In Conclusion

The ESCAPE model is based on sound principles of human behavior as well as on those of teaching and learning. It can serve as an alternative to the more rigid, rating-oriented evaluation systems. The model begins with the personal and professional values of both faculty members and students. Using the criteria-based approach, it focuses on setting meaningful and measurable objectives in the interest of helping students to grow professionally as they grapple with the increasingly complex processes, systems, procedures, and skills required in the clinical settings in which they function.

The four phases of the ESCAPE plan capitalize on the following guidelines:

1. Criticism has a negative effect on achievement of goals and objectives.

2. Praise does have some effect, one way or another, on performance.
3. Clinical performance improves most when specific mutually-set objectives are established.
4. Defensiveness resulting from critical evaluation tends to produce inferior clinical performance.
5. Coaching should be a continuing day-to-day activity. There should be no surprises at the final clinical performance evaluation conference.
6. Mutual goal setting and objective setting, not criticism, lead to improved clinical performance.
7. Clinical evaluation conferences that are designed primarily to improve students' performance should not be used as occasions to weigh promotion prospects.
8. Students' participation in the goal-setting procedure helps produce favorable results.
9. The best evaluation is self-evaluation. It can be enhanced when combined with teacher evaluation.
10. Identifying student strengths and building on them is helpful.
11. Allowing the students to contract for grades can help them set goals realistically.

For Discussion Purposes

The ESCAPE model for student clinical evaluation stands on its own yet it has some components similar to the ROPEP model for evaluating performance of nurses in hospital practice.

Imagine yourself as a member of a joint performance appraisal task force composed of representatives from both nursing education and nursing practice. The charge to the group members is to examine the potential of both appraisal models (ESCAPE and ROPEP) for contributing to identified needs and goals of the nursing profession for the next decade. The group should take into account the trends in health care generally and in its professions specifically, considering social and economic factors as well.

Compose a brief report in which you summarize the outcome of such a discussion. Be sure the report includes recommendations for how the design and use of the performance appraisal tools and techniques might be improved to better contribute to the needs and goals of nursing in both education and practice settings.

NOTES

Combs, A.S.; Avila, D.L.; & Purkey, W.W. *Helping relationships: Basic concepts for the helping profession.* Boston: Allyn & Bacon, Inc., 1971.

Ganong, J.M., & Ganong, W.L. *HELP with performance appraisal: A results-oriented approach.* Chapel Hill, N.C.: W.L. Ganong Co., 1975.

Ganong, J,M., & Ganong, W.L. *HELP with effective student clinical achievement performance evaluation.* Chapel Hill, N.C.: W.L. Ganong Co., 1977.

Ganong, J.M., & Ganong, W.L. *HELP with innovative teaching techniques.* Chapel Hill, N.C.: W.L. Ganong Co., 1979.

Ganong, J.M., & Ganong, W.L. *HELP with managerial leadership in nursing: 101 tremendous trifles* (3rd ed.). Chapel Hill, N.C.: W.L. Ganong Co., 1980.

Harvey, A. Student contracts: A break in the grading game. *Education Canada,* September 1972, p. 42.

Herzberg, F. The wise old Turk. *Harvard Business Review,* September–October 1974, *52*(5).

McCarty, P. New RN exam based on nursing process. *The American Nurse,* 1982, *14*(3).

Myers, M.S. *Every employee a manager.* New York: McGraw-Hill Book Company, 1970.

Myers, M.S. *Every employee a manager* (2nd ed.). New York: McGraw-Hill Book Company, 1981.

Raths, L.E.; Harmin, M.; & Simon, S. *Values and teaching.* Columbus, Ohio: The Charles E. Merrill Publishing Co., Inc., 1966.

Rogers, C. *Freedom to learn.* Columbus, Ohio: The Charles E. Merrill Publishing Co., Inc., 1969.

Rokeach, M. *The nature of human values.* New York: The Free Press, 1973.

Singer, B. Learning contracts: Viable alternative. *Newsletter of the Association for Humanistic Psychology,* Summer 1972.

Tosti, D. The sequential feedback model for performance assessment. In J. Springer (Ed.), *Job performance standards and measures* (Paper No. 4, ASTD Research Series). Madison, Wis.: American Society for Training & Development, 1980.

Allen Memorial Hospital

Waterloo, Iowa

246 Beds

Performance Description: Head Nurse, Nursing Service
Self-Evaluation of Performance
Criteria-Based Performance Appraisal

Reprinted by permission of Joan I. Headington, Assistant Vice President, Nursing; and John C. Omel, Vice President, Employee Services; with credit to Ellen Elsbury, Vice President, Nursing.

ALLEN MEMORIAL HOSPITAL
PERFORMANCE DESCRIPTION

TITLE: Head Nurse

DEPARTMENT: Nursing Service

I. Qualifications:
A. Graduation from an accredited school of nursing.
B. Current license in the State of Iowa.
C. Satisfactory performance in top staff nurse or charge nurse classification for a minimum of two years.
D. Demonstrated competence in management and leadership skills.
E. Ability to plan, direct, and/or implement and evaluate the nursing care delivered to a group of patients.
F. Head Nurse experience and B.S.N. degree or its equivalent preferred.

II. Position Purpose:
Coordinate management and clinical activities, in collaboration with the Area Director, on a patient unit so that optimum quality of patient care is delivered on a designated patient area consistent with the philosophy and objectives of Allen Memorial Hospital.

III. Job Relationships:
A. *Responsible to:* Area Director
B. *Supervises:* R.N., L.P.N., Nursing Assistant, Technician, Unit Secretary, & Volunteer
C. *Interrelationships:* Works effectively with the Medical Staff, other members of the health team, administrative personnel, patients, and patient families and maintains a cooperative working relationship intradepartmentally and interdepartmentally.

IV. Major Performance Responsibilities

Measures of Satisfactory Performance

Performance is satisfactory when:

A. *To Patients*
    1. Plan safe, economical, efficient, and therapeutic nurs-   JCAH, Iowa Nursing Practice Act, Minimum Standards,

IV. Major Performance Responsibilities

Measures of Satisfactory Performance

A. *To Patients* (cont'd)

ing care. Patient assignments are made according to personnel skills.

Patient Bill of Rights, Infection Control, and other relevant standards are met; and costs are controlled.

2. Help to plan and assist in patient teaching.

Patient demonstrates comprehension and performs satisfactorily. There is documentation and communication that teaching is done.

3. See that quality patient care is given to each patient in accordance with quality standards with 24-hour accountability.

Documentation on care plans and records, together with direct feedback, indicate that standards are met.

4. Give direct patient care as required.

Individual patient care needs are met, as in #3.

5. Formulate and utilize patient care plan to assist in resolving patient problems by using the Nursing Process.

Documentation on the care plan and on the patient chart indicates action on problems and progress toward discharge. Nursing diagnosis is derived from patient's status on admission and continuously thereafter. Plan is implemented, the care given is evaluated, priorities reassessed, new goals set, and plan for nursing care revised on a continuous basis.

6. Act as liaison between patient, physician, and family.

Patient and family understand and carry out physician's directions; feedback is provided to the physician.

7. Conduct nursing rounds of all patients.

At least daily nursing rounds conducted for all patients to evaluate the care being given.

8. Document on patient's chart.

Documentation reflects the care the patient is receiving and the continuing assessment of

IV. Major Performance Responsibilities	**Measures of Satisfactory Performance**
A. *To Patients* (cont'd)	
	the patient's needs, illness, response to care and treatment, pain, and general condition. Documentation is complete, factual, descriptive, accurate, and timely. All charting policies are adhered to.
9. Initiate emergency action and care when a life-threatening situation occurs (cardiac arrest, fire, tornado, adverse treatment reactions, errors, suicide attempts, etc.).	Head nurse knows exact location and proper use of emergency equipment and methods of obtaining assistance; attends B.L.S. classes; follows written policies and procedures; fills out variance reports objectively and in a timely manner.
10. Assist in quality assurance program.	Quality assurance checks are completed as assigned.
11. Assist in staffing shortages.	Assistance is provided when a staffing emergency arises.
B. *To Medical Staff*	
1. Collaborate with the physician to see that physician's orders are carried out.	Orders are carried out promptly and accurately. Qualified assistance is provided to the physician to perform examination, treatments and tests.
2. Act as liaison between physician and patient care team.	Communications are clear, as documented and used on patient care plan. Patient rounds completed with the physician.
3. Question physician when communication is not clear.	No documented errors; no negative feedback.
4. Note physician orders or delegate such.	Orders are accurate and current.

IV. Major Performance Responsibilities	Measures of Satisfactory Performance

C. *To Area Director*

1. Share appropriate communications with unit personnel.

Such communications are utilized and understood.

2. Assure adequate staffing in accordance with the matrix and patient classifications.

Personnel are assigned for adequate coverage and optimum utilization. Variation in the matrix is justified.

3. Keep Area Director informed of unit activity, personnel problems, and patients' conditions.

Appropriate information is communicated to Area Director.

4. Prepare and/or supervise patient care assignments.

Assignments are made based upon workload and competency of available personnel to meet patient care needs.

5. Seek assistance from Area Director as necessary in solving clinical and management problems.

Specific instances of seeking and using such help occur.

6. Assist Area Director with budget planning; operate unit within budget.

Budget is realistically related to patient care programs and costs are within budget. Inventory for meds, supplies, and equipment are established within budget constraints.

7. Function within the general policies, stated beliefs, and philosophy of Allen Memorial Hospital.

The hospital is represented to people with a general feeling of support and there is implementation of these policies and beliefs through both written and oral expression.

D. *To Department Personnel*

1. Act as leader, model, and innovator.

An example is set by using conferences, demonstrations, available resources, and the problem-solving method.

IV. **Major Performance Responsibilities**	**Measures of Satisfactory Performance**
D. *To Department Personnel* (cont'd)	
2. Delegate responsibilities within scope of personnel abilities	Personnel and patients' needs are met.
3. Lead regular unit personnel meetings.	Active participation is evident and there is an expression of satisfaction with unit meetings.
4. Promote an environment in which the patient care team can work cooperatively toward objectives.	Cooperative relationships exist among members of unit team.
5. Provide an opportunity for personnel staff development and provide clinical expertise.	There is evidence of participation in continuing education activities and there is a demonstration of responsibility for the teaching of personnel in areas of new techniques, changes in policies, etc.
6. Assist and monitor staff with development and usage of nursing care plans and standards of care.	Every patient care plan is current on a daily basis and follows the standard of care.
7. Monitor discharge planning, patient assignments, patient assessments, patient teaching, transfer summaries, key count, narcotic control, charts, filing of policies/procedures and SOPs, and team conferences.	All of these are current on a daily basis and accurate.
8. Counsel personnel when necessary.	Counseling is used for problem solving. A positive and constructive manner is used.
9. Evaluate personnel.	Evaluations are current and objective. Methods of improvement or disciplinary action are planned with the Area Director

IV. Major Performance Responsibilities

    D. *To Department Personnel* (cont'd)

        10. Orientation of personnel.

        11. Assistance of clinical instructors.

    E. *To Committees*

        1. Participate actively in selected committee activities.

    F. *To Other Department Personnel*

        1. Aim for intradepartmental cooperation.

        2. Keep open communication contact as needed to plan patient care.

    G. *To Other Organizations*

        1. Current membership in appropriate professional organization.

    H. *To Self*

        1. Maintain sense of personal satisfaction; keep skills up to date.

        2. Participate in continuing education and inservice programs.

Measures of Satisfactory Performance

Responsibility for the orientation and teaching of newly employed personnel and students is demonstrated.

Clinical instructors are assisted in providing students with clinical facilities, orientation, experience, and help as needed to prepare them to function as licensed nurses and/or to meet career objectives.

Committee objectives are met.

Good working relationship exists with other department personnel. Cooperation extended in lending knowledge and/or assistance to other nursing units when the need arises.

Cooperation between departments exists and favorably affects patient care.

Participation proves satisfying and productive.

Personal goals are met as related to job performance. Desired skills are kept up to date. (Refer to skills list.)

New learnings provide sense of growth and competency.

IV. Major Performance Responsibilities	Measures of Satisfactory Performance
H. *To Self* (cont'd)	
3. Demonstrate the ability to evaluate suggestions and criticisms objectively and wherever necessary undertake to change behavior or seek further guidance.	Personal responsibility shown for maintaining an unquestionable attendance and leave record.

SELF-EVALUATION OF PERFORMANCE

Name _____ Date _____

Title: _____

Department: _____ Reports to: _____

Purpose Of Your Work: (In your own words, tell the reasons for what you do.)

Performance Responsibilities: (In your own words, how well do you perform each responsibility? Include examples of results. List your response in the order as it appears on your Performance Description).

Note: Use additional sheets as necessary. When completed, return the sheet(s) to your Immediate Supervisor.

ALLEN MEMORIAL HOSPITAL
CRITERIA-BASED PERFORMANCE APPRAISAL

TITLE: <u>Head Nurse</u>

Department: <u>Nursing Service</u>

Annual: _____

Other (Explain): _____

Name _____

Unit _____ Length of time/present position _____

Period of time covered by rating: _____ to _____

Attendance Record: _____

Using the following rating scale, indicate the quality of performance by placing the appropriate letter in the block to the left of the item.

    P = Poor Quality/Performance (No criteria met)
    F = Fair Quality/Performance (Some criteria met)
    S = Satisfactory Quality/Performance (All criteria met)

The rater is expected to document his/her appraisal in the space following each item by referring to the measures of satisfactory performance as listed in the Head Nurse Performance Description.

Rating	*Items*
	I. Maintains current license to practice professional nursing in the State of Iowa. Comments:

    II. Understands the general concepts of the position purpose.
        Comments:

III. Understands the job relationships of the Head Nurse.
     Comments:

IV. Major Performance Responsibilities and Measures of Satisfactory Performance of the Head Nurse.

A. Adheres to the responsibilities to Patients.
1.   Comments:
2.
3.
4.
5.
6.
7.
8.
9.
10.
11.

B. Adheres to the responsibilities to the Medical Staff.
1.   Comments:
2.
3.
4.

C. Adheres to the responsibilities to Area Director.
1.   Comments:
2.
3.
4.
5.
6.
7.

Note: Two additional pages of this form are omitted for space reasons.

Baptist Medical Center at Columbia

Columbia, S.C.

441 Beds

Performance Evaluation—Policy and Procedure
Job Description/Performance Evaluation Form: Nurse Clinician, Nursing
Service

Reprinted with permission of Caroline N. Seigler, Vice President

PERFORMANCE EVALUATION

DEFINITION AND PURPOSE
Evaluation is a positive experience that provides an opportunity to set goals, reinforce positive behavior, correct unacceptable behavior, and provide the basis for advancement, reward, and recognition.

POLICY
1. A written evaluation will be done by the end of the probationary period (three months) and annually.
2. The evaluation should be completed, reviewed, and submitted to the Department of Human Resources at least one week prior to due date.

RESPONSIBLE PERSONS
Immediate Supervisor

EQUIPMENT/SUPPLIES
Appropriate Form

PROCEDURE

A. THREE-MONTH EVALUATION

1. Complete evaluation form and review with the employee.
2. Have employee write comments, goal, etc., and sign.
3. Review the appropriate job description/performance evaluation with the employee.
4. Submit completed evaluation to Nursing Service Office for review by appropriate person.

B. TRANSFER EVALUATION

1. Complete an evaluation when the employee transfers from one unit to another using the following guidelines:
   a. If the employee is less than six months into the evaluation year, the transferring Clinician will complete a three-month evaluation form including the employee's strengths and areas for improvement.
   b. If the employee is six months or more into the evaluation year, the transferring Clinician will complete the job description/performance evaluation and review it with the employee.

c. Review the evaluation with the employee and enter appropriate signatures.
d. Send completed form to the receiving Clinician.
e. At the time of the annual evaluation, the receiving Clinician will use the same job description/performance evaluation tool to complete the annual evaluation, entering the new date and signatures at the time of annual review.
2. Submit completed evaluations to the Nursing Service for review.

C. ANNUAL EVALUATION

1. Provide the employee the appropriate evaluation form one month prior to evaluation date.
2. Instruct the employee to provide documentation with self-evaluation (and goals).
3. Set deadline for completed self-evaluation to be returned.
4. Review anecdotal notes and other documentation in your records on the employee.
5. Review completed self-evaluation.
6. Submit completed evaluation to the Nursing Service Office for review and placement of a *Evaluation Pay Increase Authorization* form.
7. Conduct evaluation conference.
8. Retain copy of the employee's goals on the unit so that the employee can be held accountable for meeting goals.
9. Return completed evaluation to the Nursing Service Office for processing.

D. INTERNSHIP EVALUATION

1. The intern will be evaluated by the preceptor at the end of each clinical rotation.
2. Once the intern has been transferred to a permanent unit assignment, the Nurse Clinician will complete a three-month evaluation at the end of that period of time.

**BAPTIST MEDICAL CENTER AT COLUMBIA
JOB DESCRIPTION/PERFORMANCE EVALUATION**

TITLE: NURSE CLINICIAN

DEPARTMENT: Nursing Service

QUALIFICATIONS: Currently licensed as a registered nurse by the State Board of Nursing for South Carolina.

Baccalaureate degree or specific preparation in the management of patient care.

Minimum of two years' experience in nursing practice.

Demonstrated ability in coordinating the planning, implementation, and evaluation of patient care.

JOB SUMMARY: Serves as a role model for professional nurse practitioner and is responsible for utilizing skills of available nursing personnel to provide for nursing care on one unit of the hospital for sixteen (16) hours (24 hours on ICCU, ICU, L&D, Nursery, Post Partum, OR, MTU, Oncology, Psychiatry, 7 Williams, Pediatrics, Recovery Room, Emergency Department) seven (7) days a week.

SUPERVISOR: Associate Director of Nursing Services and/or Assistant Director of Nursing

Expected—Meets all of 1.0 Policies (13 criteria) plus eighty percent (80%) (64 criteria) of the expected and management-expected criteria in sections 2.0–6.0.

Above Expected—Meets all of the expected criteria (93 criteria) plus forty percent (40%) of the above-expected and management above-expected criteria (8 criteria).

Outstanding—Meets all of the expected criteria (93 criteria) plus eighty percent (80%) of the above-expected criteria (15 criteria).

Meets criteria for annual merit increase due to no disciplinary action beyond verbal counseling.

Date of Evaluation _____

Signature of Evaluator _____

Signature of Evaluatee _____

Signature of Reviewer _____

Comments: _____

_____

_____

2/79
R 10/79
R 10/81

The following performance criteria have been identified as expectations for the Nurse Clinician. All criteria are average expectations except those indicated. Circle each criterion met. Criteria unless specified are considered to be self-explanatory and met consistently. Documentation is required for all above-expected criteria. The supervisor may ask for evidence of having met other criteria.

1.0 POLICIES

Expected
1. 1 Reports to work as scheduled.
1. 2 Uses correct procedure for notification of illness.
1. 3 Completes and signs time sheet and timecard every pay period.
1. 4 Seeks approval from immediate supervisor for variations in personal work schedule.
1. 5 Wears name pin so that it is clearly visible at all times.
1. 6 Wears correct attire for area.
1. 7 Maintains personal hygiene and cleanliness.
1. 8 Knows where to locate and uses Nursing Service Manuals.
1. 9 Knows where to locate and uses Administrative Manuals.
1.10 Knows where to locate and uses other department manuals.
1.11 Conforms to Nursing Service hospital policies.
1.12 Assigns self to six (6) complete shifts as Charge Nurse per four (4)-week rotation.

1.13 Provides Nursing Service with a copy of license renewal certificate on an annual basis prior to expiration date.

2.0 NURSING PROCESS

Expected
2. 1 Utilizes assessment skills and tools to identify patient problems, needs, and interventions.
2. 2 Individualizes and maintains a written plan of care, revising as needed. Includes in care plan significant potential patient problems based on input from patient and family.
2. 3 Implements physical, psychosocial, and teaching components of patient care, identified in the care plan, according to established standards, utilizing family and interdisciplinary personnel as appropriate.
2. 4 Recognizes changes, both obvious and subtle, in signs, symptoms, and results of diagnostic studies and responds appropriately.

Management: Expected
2. 1 Assures that patients are assessed upon admission and appropriate plan of care is developed, including the physical, psychosocial, and teaching components of patient care, utilizing established standards.
2. 2 Assures that formal and informal patient care conferences are held as needed to plan or update the care of patients.
2. 3 Assures that conferences and rounds are initiated with physicians to coordinate medical and nursing plan of care.
2. 4 Assures that clinical nursing resources as well as interdisciplinary resources are utilized in individualizing the plan of care.
2. 5 Utilizes a systematic method of evaluating the quality of patient care on a weekly basis.
2. 6 Assists staff in setting priorities for action based on problem-solving process, common sense, and meeting patient care needs.
2. 7 Assures that adequate staff is posted for each tour of duty.
2. 8 Reviews previous month's time schedule and timecards for significant information regarding attendance and absences.
2. 9 Develops unit goals annually. Reviews and revises biannually and shares with immediate supervisor.
2.10 Assists with budget preparation on an annual basis.
2.11 Operates the unit within the budget on a monthly basis utilizing cost distribution and direct expense reports, etc., as evaluation tools.

2.12 Participates in and/or cooperates with projects planned by others related to nursing care.

Management: Above-Expected
2. 1 Investigates alternatives to utilization of nursing personnel for implementation of patient care.
2. 2 Implements alternatives to utilization of nursing personnel and does follow-up to evaluate effectiveness.
2. 3 Provides clinical learning experiences for nursing personnel and students to strengthen and expand clinical expertise.
2. 4 Assures that audit criteria (process or outcome), procedures, or care plans are revised or developed as needed and presented to appropriate committee.
2. 5 Utilizes personnel's work assignment to develop special abilities of individuals and meet special needs of patients.
2. 6 Plans, implements, and evaluates studies to contribute to the quality of patient care.

3.0 DOCUMENTATION OF PATIENT CARE ON PATIENT CARE RECORD

Expected
3. 1 Uses a full name and title in all signatures.
3. 2 Uses approved and appropriate abbreviations.
3. 3 Documents information in chronological order, at the time of the event or observation, with the time and date included.
3. 4 Documents and signs those events personally performed or observed.
3. 5 Documents in a clear, concise, accurate, and legible manner.
3. 6 Documents all the necessary information to communicate the patient's progress.
3. 7 Selects and initiates appropriate forms at appropriate time(s).
3. 8 Completes forms as described in charting section of Nursing Service Manuals and/or consent section of Administrative Manual.

Above-Expected
3. 1 Revises existing forms and submits to appropriate committee or resource.
3. 2 Develops new forms and submits to appropriate committee or resource.

Management-Expected
3. 1 Holds staff accountable for documentation according to Nursing Service Manuals.
3. 2 Assists with implementation of change process using new forms.
3. 3 Assists medical staff with understanding of chart forms.

4.0 CLINICAL SKILLS

Expected
4. 1 Provides personal hygiene for patient.
4. 2 Recognizes potential for skin breakdown and institutes care.
4. 3 Administers medications and parenteral therapy according to Nursing Service Manuals.
4. 4 Recognizes potential adverse symptoms to parenteral therapy and notifies physicians.
4. 5 Performs treatments and procedures according to Nursing Service Manuals.
4. 6 Utilizes skills of others in performance of treatments and procedures.
4. 7 Carries out physician's orders accurately, recognizes need for and requests changes in physician's orders, and questions unclear orders.
4. 8 Initiates nurse-physician communication regarding patient care concerns in a timely manner.
4. 9 Prepares for nurse-physician rounds by reviewing chart data.
4.10 Assists in facilitating patient-physician-nurse communication process.
4.11 Initiates and carries out appropriate emergency codes.
4.12 Maintains supplies and equipment.

Above-Expected
4. 1 Recognizes potential benefits of selected new products, and projects future supply needs in writing, and discusses with supervisor possible acquisition of use.

Management-Expected
4. 1 Serves as a role model in delivering patient care.
4. 2 Utilizes a consistent method for maintaining and controlling medications on unit.
4. 3 Critiques staff's performance during emergency codes and does follow-up.

Management Above-Expected
4. 1 Critiques performance of other personnel during emergency codes and communicates to appropriate department head.
4. 2 Participates in evaluation of new products and reports in writing to appropriate committees.

5.0 WORKING WITH OTHERS

Expected
5. 1 Maintains a positive attitude and receives no valid complaints regarding attitude or behavior.
5. 2 Identifies the need for change and possible ways of implementation in writing.
5. 3 Communicates with patients, families, unit personnel, physicians, and personnel of other departments in courteous and professional manner.
5. 4 Identifies negative feelings and discusses positive ways of dealing with those with immediate supervisor and/or other appropriate person.
5. 5 Initiates conferences in a timely manner with patients, families, unit personnel, physicians, and personnel of other departments when aware of apparent discord.
5. 6 Works effectively with unit personnel, students, instructors, and interns.

Management-Expected
5. 1 Communicates and implements change cooperatively.
5. 2 Seeks assistance from Nursing Service Administration as necessary in solving clinical and management problems.
5. 3 Informs immediate supervisor of significant unit activities, personnel problems, and patient conditions in a timely manner.
5. 4 Identifies when unit personnel need assistance and offers help.
5. 5 Maintains written anecdotal notes regarding performance of unit personnel.
5. 6 Utilizes the appropriate process for progressive discipline.
5. 7 Writes, reviews, and submits to Nursing Service Office evaluations of staff members prior to due date.
5. 8 Assists with evaluation of students as requested by instructor. Shares with instructor any problems identified in the clinical performance of the students.
5. 9 Makes self readily available to deal with individual needs and concerns of staff.

5.10 Communicates staffing needs or changes with the Assistant Director of Nursing for Staffing.

5.11 Makes self available to deal with needs and concerns of other departments as they relate to the unit.

5.12 Communicates unit needs and concerns to the Unit Manager on a regular basis.

5.13 Makes self available to discuss unit education needs with Staff Development instructor.

5.14 Makes self available to discuss patient care needs with Clinical Nurse Specialists.

5.15 Communicates appropriate changes in policies and procedures.

5.16 Shares appropriate communications with unit personnel through monthly unit meetings, communication book, clipboard, etc.

5.17 Investigates specific problems objectively and completely before making decisions.

5.18 Participates actively in administrative meetings. Reads and initials minutes when absent.

Management Above-Expected
5. 1 Assists peers with staffing or other unit problems.

5. 2 Makes self available to staff of other units in absence of Nurse Clinician.

5. 3 Gives written anecdotal notes regarding peers' performance or performance of personnel from other areas to immediate supervisor.

6.0 SELF-DEVELOPMENT

Expected
6. 1 Completes written self-evaluation according to job description one month prior to annual due date and submits to immediate supervisor. Includes goals for self-development.

6. 2 Reads selections from health care literature on a monthly basis and documents quarterly.

6. 3 Attends and participates in the Staff Development programs held at Baptist Medical Center at Columbia. Must attend all mandatory classes.

6. 4 Shares with staff information gained at hospital-sponsored workshops and documents.

6. 5 Schedules and documents periodic self-evaluation conferences with immediate supervisor to assess progress in attaining goals.

6. 6 Seeks out informal evaluation by peer groups and other members of nursing staff and documents.
6. 7 Serves as resource person for peer group.

Above-Expected
6. 1 Develops individual evaluation tools and distributes to peer group and other members of nursing staff for formal evaluation.
6. 2 Participates in the planning and/or presentation of an educational offering sponsored by Nursing Staff Development or Hospital-wide Education.
6. 3 Shares with staff information gained at workshops attended on own time and/or own expense and documents.
6. 4 Teaches or serves as a resource person using clinical expertise (hospitalwide).
6. 5 Demonstrates continued professional growth through participation in professional organizations, continuing formal education, etc.

Management-Expected
6. 1 Posts pertinent articles from health care literature on unit for staff's continuing education.
6. 2 Reviews and/or revises written unit orientation outline yearly.
6. 3 Coordinates the orientation of all new nursing personnel on unit and spends time with each new person.
6. 4 Reviews and revises as needed written guidelines for Charge Nurse on unit and reviews with staff periodically.
6. 5 Demonstrates products and equipment to staff as needed.
6. 6 Assists with identification of learning needs of staff.
6. 7 Conducts and/or coordinates at least four unit inservices per year on topics relative to needs of the unit. Documents dates held and topics.

Charlotte Rehabilitation Hospital

Charlotte, N.C.

88 Beds

Performance Descriptions:
  Charge Nurse—11–7 Shift
  Associate Nurse II
  Primary Nurse I
Employee Evaluation and Development Report

CHARLOTTE REHABILITATION HOSPITAL

TITLE: Charge Nurse—11–7 Shift

DEPARTMENT: Nursing Service

DESCRIPTION: The Charge Nurse, 11–7 shift, is a professional nurse who assumes responsibility for the patient care activities and personnel on the 11–7 shift. She also functions as an Associate Nurse and delivers direct patient care. She is responsible to the Unit Clinical Coordinators.

PERFORMANCE CRITERIA:

A. *To Self*
1. *Does self-evaluation at least annually, setting short- and long-term goals.*
   a. Documents self-evaluation and includes supporting information, anecdotals, etc.
   b. Sets time frames for goals.
   c. Identifies approaches to be used in achieving goals.
2. *Seeks out additional learning experiences, both clinically and managerially.*
   a. Attends workshops as requested, completing written report and doing oral presentation to appropriate group.
   b. Requests attendance at educational programs in appropriate manner, stating how information will be utilized.
3. *Participates in professional organization/activities.*

B. *To Patient*
1. *Assesses quality of care delivered to patients by all levels of nursing personnel assigned to the 11–7 shift.*
   a. Makes nightly rounds, observing personnel interacting with patients, and also in delivering patient care.
   b. Demonstrates care approaches to personnel as situation dictates (e.g., new personnel, new procedures, unusual requirement).
   c. Observes for compliance to established routines of care and follows through with appropriate corrective measures when routines are not followed.
2. *Functions as Associate Nurse to deliver nursing care when situation dictates.*

a. Demonstrates ability to deliver safe care and serves as role model.
b. Serves as resource to patient for identification of nursing needs.
3. *Interprets hospital/nursing service policies to patients as the need arises.*
a. Communicates policies to patients in understandable, nonbiased manner.
4. *Facilitates educational opportunities for patient by relieving Associate Nurse of unit activities.*

C. *To Associate Nurses*
1. *Assists Associate Nurses in identifying strengths, weaknesses, and providing feedback.*
a. Assesses organizational skills, direct care knowledge, and safety principles by actively participating in patient care and in direct observation.
b. Reviews flow sheet and nursing orders at least weekly.
c. Assesses Associate Nurse's utilization of bedside nursing care plan through direct observation and participation in care delivered.
d. Identifies areas of need for Associate Nurses and follows through with appropriate approaches (e.g., team conference, inservice, etc.).
e. Assists Associate Nurse (R.N.) in writing appropriate nursing orders as assessment dictates.
f. Assists Associate Nurse in understanding his/her role in the rehabilitation process, in order to help her/him follow through with appropriate feedback to Primary Nurse.
2. *Assists with orientation of new Associate Nurse.*
a. Acts as a resource person for the orientee.
b. Provides feedback, at least weekly, to Unit Clinical Coordinator on observations of performance.
c. Instructs and supervises care delivery as required (e.g., specialized procedures, those available on other units, etc.).
d. Delegates the instruction and supervision responsibilities to appropriate person in her absence.
3. *Assists Associate Nurse in dealing with patient care problems.*
a. Assists in making decision to notify attending physician or physician on call as necessary.
b. Directs emergency procedures (e.g., venipuncture, starting IV fluids, CPR) as necessary.

   c. Facilitates transfer of patient, or obtaining additional personnel
      to deliver care.
4. *Assists in performance evaluation and goal setting for the Associate
   Nurse.*
   a. Assesses performance of Associate Nurse, observing for pat-
      terns of behavior, and documentation of same.
   b. Actively participates with Unit Clinical Coordinator in evalua-
      tion conference.
   c. Provides follow-up regarding goal attainment and/or problem
      area(s) developing.

D. *To Other Nursing Personnel*
   1. *Supervises nonprofessional nursing personnel assigned to the 11–
      7 shift.*
      a. Assists in the orientation of new personnel to the 11–7 shift.
      b. Assists in teaching new procedures to personnel and communi-
         cates their abilities to the R.N.
      c. Actively participates with the Unit Clinical Coordinator in eval-
         uating their performance, and in setting goals.
      d. Provides appropriate follow-up to employee regarding goal
         attainment and/or development of problem areas.

E. *To Unit Clinical Coordinator*
   1. *Assesses the quality of the care delivered to the patients and com-
      municates this to the Unit Clinical Coordinator on the respective
      units.*
      a. Informs the Unit Clinical Coordinator within one (1) working
         day of problems and documents as necessary.
      b. Assesses problem areas identified during change of shift report
         and communicates findings to Unit Clinical Coordinator.
      c. Assesses staff's adherence to Patient Care Standards/orders,
         unit routines, and hospital policies and reports noncompliance
         patterns to Unit Clinical Coordinator.
   2. *Assists in identification of staff needs, and in setting short- and
      long-term goals in meeting the needs.*
      a. Informs Unit Clinical Coordinator(s) of needs and assists with
         formulation of approach to be used.
      b. Assists with inservice and/or follow-up on inservice for the 11–
         7 staff.
      c. Completes periodic review of procedures, routines, etc., done
         on the 11–7 shift and communicates need for further follow-up,
         if necessary.

3. *Assesses the activities on the nursing units on a daily basis and keeps Unit Clinical Coordinator(s) informed.*
   a. Reallocates staff on emergency basis, utilizing both the GRASP figures and the daily assessment.
   b. Informs Unit Clinical Coordinator(s) of changing patterns of care needs/staff performance/hospital activities that affect nursing care on 11–7 shift.
   c. Identifies areas where cost containment can be implemented.
   d. Monitors patient assignments and keeps Unit Clinical Coordinator(s) informed.

F. *To Nursing Administration* (Director of Nursing/Assistant Director)
   1. *Takes staffing call while on duty, notifying the nursing administration person on call as necessary.*
      a. Utilizes GRASP and current assessment of unit needs to guide in decision.
      b. Documents calls in appropriate manner (e.g., Payroll Information Slip, change on all time sheets).
   2. *Acts as Hospital Fire Warden until Hospital Fire Warden arrives.*
   3. *Answers all "Code Blue" calls when on duty.*
      a. Demonstrates familiarity with all emergency equipment.
      b. Directs other nursing staff present to complete required documentation, actions, etc.
      c. Restocks emergency carts after use (or leaves requisitions for the next shift and informs person in charge).
   4. *Evaluates nursing personnel as requested and documents conferences.*
      a. Evaluations are completed within the specified time frames, with any documentation/supporting statements attached.
   5. *Observes for and reports safety hazards (patient/staff/environmental).*
   6. *Actively participates in department/interdepartmental committees.*
      a. Attends 85 percent of Nursing Leadership meetings annually.
      b. Attends 75 percent of R.N./L.P.N. meetings annually.
      c. Attends other committees as appointed, at least 75 percent of time.
   7. *Does self-evaluation and sets goals at least annually, and more often, if necessary.*

QUALIFICATIONS REQUIRED:

1. Ability to work with all levels of personnel.

2. Ability to plan and organize work for self and others on one or more units.
3. Ability to adapt to new situations.
4. Ability to recognize areas of strength and weakness and to strive to develop strengths through counselling with personnel.
5. Ability to problem solve.
6. Ability to communicate needs of 11–7 staff to responsible individuals, i.e., UCC's, Assistant Director, or Director.
7. Current professional nurse registration in North Carolina.

DESIRABLE QUALIFICATIONS:

1. Experience in supervision and/or administration or growth potential with experience.
2. Leadership ability.
3. Dependability.

WORKERS SUPERVISED: Registered Nurses, Licensed Practical Nurses, R.N.A.s.

SUPERVISED BY: Unit Clinical Coordinators

PROMOTION FROM: Staff Nurse

PROMOTION TO: Unit Clinical Coordinator

REGISTERING OR LICENSING AGENCY: North Carolina Board of Nursing

---

SW
Origin: 11/71
Revised: 8/77, 8/78, 8/79, 9/81
© Charlotte Rehabilitation Hospital

TITLE: Associate Nurse II

DEPARTMENT: Nursing Service

DESCRIPTION: The Associate Nurse II is a registered professional nurse who is responsible and accountable for the direct/indirect implementation of the patient's documented care plan, in the absence of the Primary

Nurse, during his/her assigned shift. The three-shift per week day and evening R.N. and the full or part-time night R.N. will be classified as Associate II.

RESPONSIBILITIES/PERFORMANCE CRITERIA:

1. To Self:
   1.1. *Demonstrates willingness to assume some administrative responsibility.*
   1.1.a. Assumes weekend/charge nurse duties, as requested.
   1.2. *Actively participates in R.N./L.P.N. meetings and attends minimum of 75 percent of the meetings annually.*
   1.3. *Attends continuing education programs for further personal and vocational development.*
   1.4. *Attends minimum of ten (10) hours of inservice annually.*
   1.5. *Conducts periodic self-evaluation; sets goals for self at least annually.*

2. To Patients:
   2.1. *Implements directly/indirectly plan of care of assigned patients.*
   2.1.a. Gives direct patient care to assigned patients, following care plan initiated by Primary Nurse.
   2.1.b. Directs the activities of the nonprofessional personnel in giving patient care, keeping the Unit Clinical Coordinator informed as to their level of functioning.
   2.1.c. Assesses the condition of the patients assigned and suggests changes or revision of the care plan to the Primary Nurse; alters the care plan only if the condition of the patient warrants modification to meet immediate needs.
   2.2. *Documents information relevant to patients assigned.*
   2.2.a. Records pertinent information on appropriate flow sheets daily.
   2.2.b. Updates nursing care plan as indicated, in the absence of Primary Nurse.
   2.2.c. Updates PCU as needed in absence of Primary Nurse.
   2.3. *Delivers safe nursing care.*
   2.3.a. Administers prescribed medications, orally and by injection.
   2.2.b. Accurately transcribes and executes physicians' orders in conformance with established procedures.
   2.2.c. Identifies and removes (if possible) environmental hazards or refers to appropriate persons for action.

3. To Primary Nurse:
   3.1. *Communicates with Primary Nurse on continuous basis.*
      3.1.a. Utilizes taped, oral, written report or combination of these on a regular basis.
      3.1.b. Writes SOAP note in the absence of the Primary Nurse.
      3.1.c. Informs Unit Clinical Coordinator of the change in patient status in the absence of the Primary Nurse (Evening Supervisor, Night Charge Nurse on those shifts).
   3.2. *Attends conferences in the absence of the Primary Nurse.*
      3.2.a. Actively participates in the conferences when representing the Primary Nurse.
      3.2.b. Communicates outcome of conferences of Primary Nurse and peers, in timely manner.
   3.3. *Assists the Primary Nurse in providing family/patient teaching.*
      3.3.a. Assists the Primary Nurse in identifying the patient/family needs for information and helps provide opportunities for instruction.
      3.3.b. Assists the Primary Nurse in providing opportunities for the patient/family to have direct involvement in care, providing feedback to the Primary Nurse on the progress made.
      3.3.c. Assists the Primary Nurse in assessing the ability of the patient/family to perform the required tasks.

4. To Physician:
   4.1. *Makes rounds with physicians.*
      4.1.a. Makes rounds with physician in the absence of the Primary Nurse; communicates this information to Primary Nurse and/or Unit Clinical Coordinator.
      4.1.b. Accurately writes any necessary verbal orders that may result from rounds.

5. To Other Nursing Personnel:
   5.1. *Actively participates in the evaluation of the L.P.N. and nonprofessional nursing personnel.*
      5.1.a. Assists in making and implementing recommendations for improving performance.
      5.1.b. Documents strengths and weaknesses observed in appropriate manner.
   5.2. *Participates in orientation of new personnel and in evaluating their performance.*
   5.3. *Assists in identifying individual needs of staff, participates in on-the-spot teaching, and communicates to appropriate person(s) areas of need.*

6. To Others: (Health Team Members)

    6.1. *Collaborates with health team members in facilitating working relationships that result in a smoothly functioning environment.*

    6.2. *Demonstrates willingness to compromise with other health team members appropriately as situation dictates, to ensure quality patient care.*

QUALIFICATIONS REQUIRED:

1. Current professional nurse registration in North Carolina.
2. Demonstrated ability to administer safe nursing care.
3. Adequate knowledge of both normal and abnormal anatomy, physiology, psycho/social, and disease entities.
4. Ability to initiate and implement all phases of the nursing process.
5. Ability to communicate effectively with others involved in patient care.
6. Ability to utilize effective teaching methods in relating to patients, families, and staff members.
7. Ability to work with others, both supervisors and subordinates.

DESIRABLE QUALIFICATIONS:

1. Working knowledge of philosophy and principles of rehabilitative nursing.
2. Good mental and physical health.
3. Leadership ability.
4. Ability to problem solve.
5. Demonstrated interest in professional growth and development.
6. Working knowledge of philosophy and principles of primary nursing.
7. Working knowledge of Problem-Oriented Medical Record.

WORKERS SUPERVISED:
Licensed Practical Nurses and auxiliary nursing personnel of unit.

SUPERVISED BY:
Unit Clinical Coordinator

PROMOTION FROM:
No formal line of promotion

PROMOTION TO:
Primary Nurse I or II

REGISTERING OR LICENSING AGENCY:
North Carolina Board of Nursing

SW
Origin: 12/77
Revised: 11/79, 4/80, 1/81, 2/82, 11/82
NSG. 72 Page 3
© Charlotte Rehabilitation Hospital

TITLE: Primary Nurse I

DEPARTMENT: Nursing Service

DESCRIPTION: The Primary Nurse I is a registered professional nurse who has previous rehabilitative nursing experience and is in his/her 90-day probationary period, or a nurse who is in his/her first year of rehabilitative nursing experience. He/she is responsible and accountable for the direct and/or indirect rehabilitative nursing care of a limited number of patients assigned to him/her, from the time of admission to discharge. This is an entry-level position.

RESPONSIBILITIES/PERFORMANCE CRITERIA:

1. To Self:
    1.1. *Recognizes limitations and seeks appropriate resource person when necessary.*
    1.2. *Actively participates in R.N./L.P.N. meetings and attends minimum of 75 percent of the meetings annually.*
    1.3. *Attends continuing education programs for further personal and vocational development.*
    1.4. *Attends minimum of ten (10) hours of approved inservice annually.*
    1.5. *Conducts periodic self-evaluation; sets goals for self at least annually.*

2. To Patients:
    2.1. *Initiates and implements all phases of the nursing process.*
        2.1.a. Completes admission assessment of new patient within 2 to 3 hours of admission, with assistance.
        2.1.b. Writes initial, basic nursing orders on the day of admission with assistance.
        2.1.c. Initiates problems and goals sheet, writes nursing orders, (plan of care) within 48 hours, and updates as indicated.

2.1.d. Completes UR information, basic nursing equipment list, and PCU information, on the day of admission, with assistance.
2.1.e. Implements and/or directs plan of care, with assistance.
2.1.f. Reassesses the patients' needs and plan of care daily, revising as necessary.
2.2. *Documents all information relevant to patient care.*
   2.2.a. Records pertinent observations on nursing activity flow sheet(s).
   2.2.b. Completes initial nursing problems and goals form, within 48 hours of admission, with assistance.
   2.2.c. Writes SOAP note as often as necessary, indicating goal attainment, lack of attainment, change of time frame/goals, with assistance.
   2.2.d. Documents patient/family teaching appropriately.
   2.2.e. Completes discharge form within week prior to discharge.
2.3. *Participates actively in patient care, as well as direct care received by patient in her/his absence, via Nursing Care Plan.*
   2.3.a. Gives direct care to both primary and associate patients.
   2.3.b. Assumes responsibility for and directs care to be given in his/her absence via clearly defined written nursing care plan.
2.4. *Provides patient/family teaching.*
   2.4.a. Identifies patient/family basic care teaching needs and provides opportunities for formal and informal instruction.
   2.4.b. Provides patient/family with appropriate pamphlets or books as needed to reinforce teaching program.
   2.4.c. Provides opportunities to participate in direct care activities, as under supervision and independently, in preparation for discharge, and communicates outcomes to team members appropriately.
   2.4.d. Begins to assume responsibility for assessing patient/family to perform required tasks, documents, and makes referral when their achievement of tasks is questionable.
2.5. *Actively participates in discharge planning.*
   2.5.a. Participates in discharge planning meeting.
   2.5.b. Identifies any unmet goals for discharge and communicates to appropriate person.
   2.5.c. Obtains prescriptions; does appropriate teaching.
2.6. *Delivers safe nursing care.*
   2.6.a. Demonstrates priority setting in care delivery.
   2.6.b. Follows approved prescribed policies and procedures.

2.6.c. Administers prescribed medication, orally and by injection.
2.6.d. Directs activities of auxiliary personnel in rendering direct/indirect care.
2.6.e. Accurately transcribes and executes M.D. orders, in conformance with proper technique and established procedures.
2.6.f. Identifies and removes (if possible) environmental hazards or refers to appropriate persons for action.

3. To Associate Nurse
   3.1. *Communicates patients' needs and progress to Associate Nurse.*
      3.1.a. Observes and communicates significant information through appropriate channels.
      3.1.b. Consults with peers and other disciplines when appropriate.

4. To Physician
   4.1. *Makes rounds with physicians.*
      4.1.a. Communicates appropriate information to physician.
      4.1.b. Requests orders as needed, in timely manner.

5. To Others (Health Team Members)
   5.1. *Begins to collaborate with health team members in implementing total rehabilitation program.*

QUALIFICATIONS REQUIRED:

1. Current professional nurse registration in North Carolina.
2. Demonstrated ability to administer safe nursing care.
3. Adequate knowledge of both normal and abnormal anatomy, physiology, psycho/social, and disease entities.
4. Ability to initiate and implement all phases of the nursing process.
5. Ability to communicate effectively with others involved in patient care.
6. Ability to work with others, both supervisors and subordinates.

DESIRABLE QUALIFICATIONS:

1. Working knowledge of philosophy and principles of rehabilitative nursing.
2. Good mental and physical health.
3. Leadership ability.
4. Ability to problem solve.
5. Demonstrated interest in professional growth and development.

6. Working knowledge of philosophy and principles of primary nursing.
7. Working knowledge of Problem-Oriented Medical Record.

WORKERS SUPERVISED:
Licensed Practical Nurses and auxiliary nursing personnel of unit.

SUPERVISED BY:
Unit Clinical Coordinator

PROMOTION FROM:
No formal line of promotion.

PROMOTION TO:
Primary Nurse II

REGISTERING OR LICENSING AGENCY:
North Carolina Board of Nursing

Origin: 12/77
Revised: 11/79, 1/81, 2/82, 11/82
Nsing. 17 Page 3
© Charlotte Rehabilitation Hospital

CHARLOTTE REHABILITATION HOSPITAL
EMPLOYEE EVALUATION AND DEVELOPMENT REPORT

NAME _____ ANNIVERSARY DATE _____

POSITION _____ SHIFT _____

DAYS ABSENT _____ SICK _____ LOA _____

EDUCATIONAL PROGRAMS ATTENDED _____

MERIT INCREASE REQUESTED YES _____ NO _____

RE-EVALUATION DATE _____

GENERAL INSTRUCTIONS FOR USE OF CRITERIA-BASED EVALUATION:

The criteria-based evaluation form is to be completed at the end of the 90-day probationary period and at the first anniversary, then annually thereafter unless otherwise indicated above.

If "yes" is checked, there must be evidence that the criterion is met 85% of the time. If "no" is checked, there must be substantiating comments written in the space provided. If the criterion does not apply (e.g., because of shift assignment) write "N/A." In the space provided for comments, please identify the specific criterion being commented upon.

Perf. Criteria   COMMENTS

No.	Yes/No		
____	____	____	_____
____	____	____	_____
____	____	____	_____
____	____	____	_____
____	____	____	_____
____	____	____	_____
____	____	____	_____
____	____	____	_____
____	____	____	_____
____	____	____	_____
____	____	____	_____
____	____	____	_____
____	____	____	_____
____	____	____	_____
____	____	____	_____
____	____	____	_____
____	____	____	_____
____	____	____	_____
____	____	____	_____
____	____	____	_____
____	____	____	_____
____	____	____	_____
____	____	____	_____
____	____	____	_____
____	____	____	_____
____	____	____	_____
____	____	____	_____
____	____	____	_____
____	____	____	_____
____	____	____	_____
____	____	____	_____
____	____	____	_____
____	____	____	_____

Perf. Criteria   COMMENTS

No.	Yes/No		
___	___	___	_____
___	___	___	_____
___	___	___	_____
___	___	___	_____
___	___	___	_____
___	___	___	_____
___	___	___	_____
___	___	___	_____
___	___	___	_____
___	___	___	_____
___	___	___	_____
___	___	___	_____
___	___	___	_____
___	___	___	_____
___	___	___	_____
___	___	___	_____
___	___	___	_____
___	___	___	_____
___	___	___	_____
___	___	___	_____
___	___	___	_____
___	___	___	_____
___	___	___	_____
___	___	___	_____
___	___	___	_____
___	___	___	_____
___	___	___	_____
___	___	___	_____
___	___	___	_____
___	___	___	_____
___	___	___	_____

GOALS (Describe any goals or expected improvements for the coming year.)

_____

_____

_____

EMPLOYEE COMMENTS: _____

_____

_____

_____

_____

_____   _____
EMPLOYEE SIGNATURE   DATE

_____   _____
SUPERVISOR SIGNATURE   DATE

5/80 Nsg. Trial Form

Jenkins Methodist Home

Watertown, S.D.

Job Performance Standards:
  Nurse Aide
  Licensed Practical Nurse
  Registered Nurse

_____

Reprinted by permission of Mary Cordell, Director of Nursing Service

JENKINS METHODIST HOME, INC.

JOB PERFORMANCE STANDARDS
NURSE AIDE

Brief Job Summary: Works under the supervision and guidance of a professional staff nurse; is involved in providing daily services involving basic resident care.

I. Major Performance Responsibilities —	4 Superior	3 Above Avg.	2 Satisfactory	1 Needs Improving
1. Handling and serving residents in safe and comfortable manner: by using correct medical asepsis; provides for residents protection; prevents hazards of immobility.				
2. Adhering to instruction issued by supervising nurse.				
3. Performing duties established by nursing policies and routine procedures: by assisting residents with personal care; providing nutrition and fluids; assisting residents in elimination needs.				
4. Maintaining good housekeeping standards within assigned duty areas.				
5. Ability to see and do (complete) tasks not already assigned.				
6. Able to organize work so that it can be completed on time.				
7. Shares appropriate communications with co-workers and community representatives.				
8. Keeps supervising nurse informed of requests/changes in residents condition.				
9. Cleans and handles equipment as assigned.				
10. Faithfulness in coming to work and conforming to work hours as scheduled.				
11. Ability to accept criticism — works smoothly with and for others.				
12. Communicates effectively with patients.				
13. Ability to adjust to changing situations and work assignments.				
14. Usually well-groomed, neat and in appropriate uniform.				
15. TOTAL SCORE				

II. Supervisor please outline specific strengths, problems, weak areas.

_____

_____

_____

_____

Form 47-P.O.-1M-9-80

JENKINS METHODIST HOME, INC.

NAME _____

TO BE COMPLETED BY AIDE:

You can help prepare an up-to-date performance description of what you do in your work. Please answer the following as complete as possible.

1. The purpose of my work is:

_____

_____

2. How do you know whether or not you are performing your work satisfactorily?

_____

_____

3. List anything which you think should NOT be a part of your work.

_____

_____

4. List anything you are NOT doing which YOU think SHOULD BE a part of your work.

_____

_____

5. Comments and suggestions — anything else that will help your work and how you feel about it.

_____

_____

_____

_____

6. I agree/do not agree with the above evaluation . . .

_____

_____

_____

Employee's Signature _____ Date _____

Supervisor's Signature _____ Date _____

Rating — To be completed by Director of Nursing _____

Signature _____ Date _____

Form 50-P.O. 1M-9-80

JENKINS METHODIST HOME, INC.

JOB PERFORMANCE STANDARDS
LPN

Brief Job Summary: Renders professional nursing care to residents within an assigned unit. Plans resident care; coordinates staff activities; implements resident care; evaluates resident care.

	4 Superior	3 Above Avg.	2 Satisfactory	1 Needs Improving
1. Demonstrates awareness of the comprehensive nature of long-term care.				
2. Gives direct resident care when needed. Has developed nursing skills of an acceptable level of competency in accordance with educational level.				
3. Makes nursing rounds to assess resident needs.				
4. Helps develop nursing care plans to meet on-going Needs/Problems/Concerns requests of residents.				
5. Acts as a liaison between resident, physician, family and community.				
6. Discusses resident care goals with physician during rounds.				
7. Prepares both written and oral reports regarding resident symptoms, reaction, changes and requests, and reports to attending physician.				
8. Questions physician when communication is not clear.				
9. Takes responsibility for carrying out physician's orders.				
10. Assists physician with rounds, treatments, and diagnostic procedures.				
11. Provides adequate communication with staff by making out resident care assignments.				
12. Assesses resident care given by staff and implements appropriate changes.				
13. Functions as leader, innovator, holds regular floor meetings.				
14. Performs duties in accordance with established policy and procedures.				
15. Promotes open communication within nursing unit between co-workers, residents, family, and community.				
16. Promotes open communication between department head, co-workers, residents, family, and community.				

Form 52-P.O.-1M-9-80

JOB PERFORMANCE STANDARDS: (CONT.)

	4 Superior	3 Above Avg.	2 Satisfactory	1 Needs Improving
17. Attends scheduled staff meetings regularly.				
18. Adaptable in changing situations and work assignments.				
19. Participates in selected committees to promote quality resident care.				
20. Maintains a sense of personal satisfaction by showing willingness to update nursing skills.				
21. Participates in in-service and continuing education when offered by facility.				
22. Promotes open communication to other departments as needed to plan resident care.				
23. Ability to accept criticism — works smoothly with and for others.				
24. Usually well groomed — neat and in appropriate uniform.				
25. TOTAL SCORE				

26. Specific strengths, problems, weak areas:

_____

_____

_____

_____

_____

27. My goals are:

_____

_____

_____

_____

_____

_____

JENKINS METHODIST HOME, INC.

JOB PERFORMANCE STANDARDS
RN

Brief Job Summary: Renders professional nursing care to residents within an assigned unit. Is accountable for demonstrating ability to identify and utilize biological, psysiological, behavioral and sociological assessment principles necessary for quality resident care. Plans, implements, evaluates care, coordinates staff activities.

	4 Superior	3 Above Avg.	2 Satisfactory	1 Needs Improving
1. Demonstrates awareness of the comprehensive nature of long-term care.				
2. Gives direct resident care when needed. Has developed nursing skills of an acceptable level of competency in accordance with educational level.				
3. Makes nursing rounds to assess resident needs.				
4. Helps develop nursing care plans to meet on-going Needs/Problems/Concerns requests of residents.				
5. Acts as a liaison between resident, physician, family and community.				
6. Discusses resident care goals with physician during rounds.				
7. Prepares both written and oral reports regarding resident symptoms, reaction, changes and requests; and reports to attending physician.				
8. Questions physician when communication is not clear.				
9. Takes responsibility for carrying out physician's orders.				
10. Assists physician with rounds, treatments, and diagnostic procedures.				
11. Provides adequate communication with staff by making out resident care assignments.				
12. Assesses resident care given by staff and implements appropriate changes.				
13. Functions as leader, innovator, holds regular floor meetings.				
14. Performs duties in accordance with established policy and procedures.				
15. Promotes open communication within nursing unit between co-workers, residents, family, and community.				
16. Promotes open communication between department head, co-workers, residents, family, and community.				

Form SLP.0. 1M 9/80

JOB PERFORMANCE STANDARDS: (CONT.)

	4 Superior	3 Above Avg.	2 Satisfactory	1 Needs Improving
17. Attends scheduled staff meetings regularly.				
18. Adaptable in changing situations and work assignments.				
19. Participates in selected committees to promote quality resident care.				
20. Maintains a sense of personal satisfaction by showing willingness to update nursing skills.				
21. Participates in in-service and continuing education when offered by facility.				
22. Promotes open communication to other departments as needed to plan resident care.				
23. Ability to accept criticism — works smoothly with and for others.				
24. Usually well-groomed — neat and in appropriate uniform.				
25. Ability to identify and discriminate between physical and psychological signs/symptoms essential to the effective management and planning of resident care.				
26. Ability to assess and provide preventative, restorative and supportive resident care.				
27. Involvement in health teaching to staff and resident, necessary for promotion of quality resident care.				
28. Responsible and accountable for biological, physiological, behavioral and sociological assessment principles necessary for competent resident care planning.				
29. TOTAL SCORE				

30. Specific strengths, problems, weak areas:

_____

_____

_____

31. My goals are:

_____

_____

_____

JENKINS METHODIST HOME, INC.

NAME _____

TO BE COMPLETED BY RN OR LPN:
You can help prepare an up-to-date performance description of what you do in your work. Please answer the following as completely as possible.

1. Select one of the job standards you are not in full agreement with as stated and rewrite it with your own idea of how to measure satisfactory performance.

_____

_____

_____

_____

2. Complete the following statement: I feel we need to improve on the following . . .

_____

_____

_____

_____

3. I understand/do not understand my job performance standards but would like to comment on the following . . .

_____

_____

_____

_____

4. I agree/do not agree with my evaluation . . .

_____

_____

Employee's Signature _____ Date _____

Rating — To be done by Director of Nursing _____

Signature _____ Date _____

Form 49 P.O. 250 9 80

Johnston-Willis Hospital

Richmond, Va.

252 Beds

Performance Appraisal System Evaluation Form:
Head Nurse

PERFORMANCE APPRAISAL SYSTEM FOR HEAD NURSES

1. The performance appraisal shall be completed by the Supervisor and reviewed by the Director/Assistant Director of Nursing.

2. The Head Nurse shall complete performance appraisal for herself/himself.

3. After completing the above steps, a conference will be scheduled and a permanent performance appraisal will be developed from this conference.

4. The permanent form will be forwarded to the Personnel Department and a copy will be kept by the Director and will be available to the Supervisor. A copy of the summary and developmental sheet will be given to the Head Nurse.

5. Evaluations will be conducted at regular intervals as specified in the Employee Handbook, and more often if needed.

JOHNSTON-WILLIS HOSPITAL
PERFORMANCE APPRAISAL

Job Title: Head Nurse   Employee_____

Department: Nursing   Evaluator_____

Reports: Nursing Supervisor

Supervises: Registered Nurses, Licensed Practical Nurses, Nursing Attendants,
                Nursing Assistants, Ward Clerks, Private Duty Nurses, Nursing
                Students and Volunteers.

Job Summary: To plan, organize by setting goals and objectives, and direct all
                unit activities by assuming responsibility for the complete nurs-
                ing care given on the patient care unit. In addition, to evaluate
                the effectiveness of the staff and unit performance, and coordi-
                nate the unit activities with other departments.

Instructions: Evaluation form shall be completed by the Nursing Supervisor and
                shall be reviewed by the Director/Assistant Director of Nursing.
                Both employee and evaluator are invited to write in the "Comments"
                sections.

                Circle the number that best represents your answer.

PERFORMANCE DEFINITIONS

5.) Exceptional Performance   Highest rating for performance reserved
                                     for those individuals whose results
                                     achieved were exceptional and who con-
                                     tinually utilize their abilities in a
                                     manner which is rarely equaled.

4.) Exceeds Requirements   Performance continually exceeds normal
                                     expectations and job requirements.

3.) Meets Requirements   Performance consistently meets normal
                                     expectations and job requirements.

2.) Meets Most Requirements   Performance does not consistently meet
                                     normal expectations and job requirements,
                                     improvement is expected.

1.) Fails To Meet Requirements   Performance failed to meet normal expec-
                                     tations and job requirements.

NOTE TO EVALUATORS: Any rating lower than "3" MUST be accompanied by a
                     justifying comment.

PERFORMANCE RESPONSIBILITIES	EVALUATION CRITERIA

Responsibilities To The Patient:

1.a. Supervise patient care to make sure that all patients receive optimum care.

   b. Make rounds to assess any patient needs.

   c. Make rounds to assess staff accomplishments and what immediate needs are still to be met.

1.a. Supervisor and Head Nurse will meet at least once daily to discuss clinical problems on the patient care unit.

   b. Daily patient rounds are made. No patient complaints of inadequate care are received.

   c. Overtime is maintained within the range of the hospital objective.

1   2   3   4   5

Comments:_____
_____
_____
_____

2. Assure that an individualized nursing care plan is provided for each patient.

2. Any deficiencies in nursing care plans are noted at least daily.

1   2   3   4   5

Comments:_____
_____
_____
_____

3. Assure that the kardex is checked with medex on each shift.

3. Supervisor reviews documentation sheet attached to medex to see there are no discrepancies or discrepancies are corrected.

1   2   3   4   5

Comments:_____
_____
_____
_____

PERFORMANCE RESPONSIBILITIES	EVALUATION CRITERIA

Responsibilities To The Patient:

4. Maintain emergency equipment and unit supplies at a set inventory.

4. Standard is met when there are no reports to Supervisor of inadequate supplies.

1   2   3   4   5

Comments:_____

5. Assure that the patient's educational needs are recognized and met.

5. Kardex and Discharge Summary Sheet will reflect that this has been done.

1   2   3   4   5

Comments:_____

6. Assure that adequate discharge planning takes place for all patients and their families.

6. Discharge forms will be periodically reviewed by the Head Nurse or designee to see that this task has been completed.

1   2   3   4   5

Comments:_____

7. Assist all staff to maintain safe equipment and environment.

7. No reported accidents caused by unsafe environment.

1   2   3   4   5

Comments:_____

PERFORMANCE RESPONSIBILITIES	EVALUATION CRITERIA

Responsibilities Patient's Families:

8. Communicate with and reassure families.

8. No problems indicated by families caused by inadequate information.

1   2   3   4   5

Comments:_____
_____
_____

9. Supervise, assist, and evaluate the patient care provided by private duty nurses.

9.a. Head Nurse meets with private duty nurse and reports any problems to Supervisor.

b. Head Nurse assures that an evaluation of the private duty nurse is completed upon the termination of the nurse's care for the patient. (Documented.)

1   2   3   4   5

Comments:_____
_____
_____

Responsibilities To The Physician:

10. Assure that all pertinent nursing information is documented on the medical record.

10. Documentation deficiencies reported by the Nursing Quality Assurance Committee are investigated by the Head Nurse and appropriate action taken.

1   2   3   4   5

Comments:_____
_____
_____

PERFORMANCE RESPONSIBILITIES	EVALUATION CRITERIA

Responsibilities To The Physician: (Continued)

11. Responsible to see that all pertinent patient information is communicated to the physician.

11. Head Nurse will verbally respond to physician questions concerning patient progress or seek out the information and report this daily.

1　　2　　3　　4　　5

Comments:_____

_____

_____

12. Completes patient rounds with the physician or delegates this responsibility.

12. Verbal reports are given to Supervisor indicating any physician complaints about lack of nurse attendance during rounds.

1　　2　　3　　4　　5

Comments:_____

_____

_____

13. Assure that physician's orders are carried out correctly and promptly.

13. No incident reports or negative feedback from physician.

1　　2　　3　　4　　5

Comments:_____

_____

_____

14. Arrange the orderly transfer of patients as indicated in adherence to established transfer

14. No complaints from patient's families and physicians about patient's transfer, and no transfer procedure deficiencies.

1　　2　　3　　4　　5

Comments:_____

_____

_____

PERFORMANCE RESPONSIBILITIES	EVALUATION CRITERIA

Responsibilities To The Unit Staff:

15. Plan adequate coverage for each 24 hour period of the four-week work schedule.

    15. Supervisor will receive and approve the four-week work schedule two weeks prior to its use.

      1   2   3   4   5

      Comments:_____

16. Assign and assure that staff attend scheduled inservice programs and staff or committee meetings.

    16. No deficiencies in staff attendance reported by Staff Development on a program-by-program basis.

      1   2   3   4   5

      Comments:_____

17. Organize nursing teams, designate a charge nurse, or team leader and evaluate team effectiveness.

    17. Head Nurse will review on a regular basis nursing team assignments and observe team effectiveness.

      1   2   3   4   5

      Comments:_____

18. Hold staff conferences at least once a month and keep a record of attendance and content.

    18. Head Nurse will hold staff team conferences at least once per month and document attendance and content.

      1   2   3   4   5

      Comments:_____

PERFORMANCE RESPONSIBILITIES	EVALUATION CRITERIA

Responsibilities To The Unit Staff: (Continued)

19. Maintain the continuity of pa-
    tient care during the patient's
    assignment to the unit.

19. Head Nurse insures that effective
    reporting, nursing notes and up-
    dated care plans are kept and e-
    valuated by absence of incidents
    due to lack of information.

    1   2   3   4   5

    Comments:_____
    _____
    _____
    _____

20. Communicate with members of the
    staff concerning new policies
    and procedures and inform them
    of changes in existing policies
    and procedures.

20. One of these communication tools
    will document instruction on new
    changes in policy and procedure:

    a. Unit Log.
    b. Wonder Board.
    c. Staff Meeting Minutes.
    d. Head Nurse Council Minutes.

    1   2   3   4   5

    Comments:_____
    _____
    _____
    _____

21. Serve as resource person to unit
    staff members.

21. No reports to or observations by
    Supervisor of lack of assistance
    from Head Nurse.

    1   2   3   4   5

    Comments:_____
    _____
    _____
    _____

PERFORMANCE RESPONSIBILITIES	EVALUATION CRITERIA

Responsibilities To The Unit Staff: (Continued)

22. Conduct performance evaluations for unit staff members.

22. Responsibility is accomplished when completed evaluations are forwarded to appropriate Supervisor by the anniversary date.

1   2   3   4   5

Comments:_____
_____
_____
_____

23. Council with staff members and document the conference content in employee's file. Recommend discipline, transfer, promotion, and termination of employees.

23. Progress Notes indicate counseling performed, employee grievances dealt with, and staff conflicts addressed.

1   2   3   4   5

Comments:_____
_____
_____
_____

24. Assist in the interviewing and hiring of prospective employees.

24. Written assessment summary is returned to recruiter within 24 hours after interview.

1   2   3   4   5

Comments:_____
_____
_____
_____

25. Provide for the orientation of new personnel.

25. Orientation checklist is completed and filed in each employee's folder within two months of the employee's anniversary date.

1   2   3   4   5

Comments:_____
_____
_____
_____

PERFORMANCE RESPONSIBILITIES	EVALUATION CRITERIA

Responsibilities To The Nursing Student:

26. Assist in the provision of clinical experiences for students of affiliating schools.

26. No student or instructor reports a lack of help provided by the Head Nurse.

   1   2   3   4   5

Comments: _____

Responsibilities To The Supervisors:

27. Provide Supervisors with necessary information concerning: unit activities; unusual incidents; needs and problems of patients and personnel.

27. Supervisor is informed daily concerning unit needs and problems.

   1   2   3   4   5

Comments: _____

Responsibilities To The Department:

28. Attend Head Nurse Council Meetings and other assigned committee meetings or scheduled meetings.

28. Attends 90% of each committee assigned and other scheduled meetings and actively participates.

   1   2   3   4   5

Comments: _____

29. Assist in the development of the yearly departmental budgets.

29. Provides all necessary information, follows established procedures and meets established time deadlines.

   1   2   3   4   5

Comments: _____

PERFORMANCE RESPONSIBILITIES	EVALUATION CRITERIA

Responsibilities To Other Departments:

30. Coordinate patient activities and unit needs with other departments.

30. No significant reports from other departments about lack of cooperation from the Head Nurse.

1　　　　2　　　　3　　　　4　　　　5

Comments:_____
_____
_____
_____

Responsibilities To The Hospital:

31. Maintain adequate communication with rescue squads, ambulance services, and outside agencies.

31. No reported problems.

1　　　　2　　　　3　　　　4　　　　5

Comments:_____
_____
_____
_____

32. Communicate all pertinent information to nursing and/or hospital administration.

32. Director and Administrator are informed as problems arise.

1　　　　2　　　　3　　　　4　　　　5

Comments:_____
_____
_____
_____

33. Adhere to established policies of the hospital and department.

33. No reported incidents as a result of a lack of conformance to established policies.

1　　　　2　　　　3　　　　4　　　　5

Comments:_____
_____
_____
_____

PERFORMANCE RESPONSIBILITIES	EVALUATION CRITERIA

Responsibilities To The Hospital: (Continued)

34. Assist unit personnel in completing annual physical examinations on a timely basis.

34. No deficiencies indicated by reports from Employee Health.

    1   2   3   4   5

    Comments:_____

35. Assist in accounting for all chargeable items, supplies, equipment, and IV materials.

35. No deficiencies indicated by reports from Materiels Management and or Pharmacy.

    1   2   3   4   5

    Comments:_____

36. Conduct investigations for incident reports as necessary.

36. Within 24 hours of incident, prepare a report and offer suggestions for prevention of similar incidents

    1   2   3   4   5

    Comments:_____

37. Assist the evaluation of products and equipment.

37. Demonstrates that responsibility is carried out by the completion of the evaluation form within the specified time frame.

    1   2   3   4   5

    Comments:_____

PERFORMANCE RESPONSIBILITIES	EVALUATION CRITERIA

Responsibilities To Herself:

38. Attend inservice and continuing education programs and courses.

38. Staff Development records will indicate whether or not Head Nurse attends 80% of inservice education programs.

1	2	3	4	5

Comments:_____
_____
_____
_____

39. Present annual report on new information gained at a workshop or through individual study to a group of one's colleagues.

39. Head Nurse presents an annual report to colleagues on new information gained from workshop attendance or individual study.

1	2	3	4	5

Comments:_____
_____
_____
_____

40. Complete an annual physical examination on a timely basis and maintain good health.

40. Have annual physical exam on time from Employee Health.

1	2	3	4	5

Comments:_____
_____
_____
_____

SUMMARY AND DEVELOPMENTAL SHEET

EMPLOYEE STRENGTHS: _____
_____
_____
_____

DEVELOPMENT AREAS: _____
_____
_____
_____

DEVELOPMENTAL PROGRAM		
PROJECTED DATE OF COMPLETION	ACTIVITY	ACTUAL DATE OF COMPLETION

COMMENTS OF SUPERVISOR: _____
_____

COMMENTS OF EMPLOYEE: _____
_____

ACKNOWLEDGEMENT OF DISCUSSION AND REVIEW

The contents of this review have been discussed with me by my supervisor, and I am fully aware of this information.

_____
Employee's Signature

_____
Date

I have discussed the contents of this review with the employee on

_____
Supervisor's Signature

Reviewed by   Date

(1/82)

Loma Linda University Medical Center

Loma Linda, Calif.

494 Beds

Background
Diagram: Clinical/Administrative Ladder
Qualification and Job Summaries
Job Descriptions:
    Clinical Nurse I
    Clinical Nurse II
    Clinical Nurse III
    Clinical Nurse IV
Nurse Practice Expectations and Evaluation:
    Clinical Nurse I
    Clinical Nurse II

Reprinted by permission of Job Description Committee, Marilyn Thungquest, Chairman, Nursing Division, and Gertrude Haussler, Vice President.

ABOUT OUR ORGANIZATION

Loma Linda University Medical Center is affiliated with the Seventh-day Adventist Church and with Loma Linda University's schools of nursing, medicine, dentistry, allied health professions, and public health. The Medical Center is a nonprofit, tertiary care facility that accepts patients from roughly one-quarter of California. The Medical Center's motto, "To Make Man Whole," reflects the commitment of the professionals practicing here to minister to the body, mind, and spirit of patients and their families.

The Division of Nursing at Loma Linda University Medical Center is organized into six clinical departments (parent/child, surgical, medical, critical care, emergency, and special services) and one education department. Incorporated into the Division's philosophy is the idea that coordinated patient care reduces fragmentation and duplication. Nurses are well prepared to provide such coordination. We believe interdisciplinary collaboration improves patient care and soon will be implementing a form for multidisciplinary care planning.

INTRODUCTION TO THE SERIES

The Nursing Job Description Committee was appointed to develop a "clinical ladder" for nursing functions: a sequence of progressively more responsible nursing levels. The clinical ladder incorporates the following ideas:

1. The knowledge and skills of the expert nurse are reflected in the job description.
2. Assignment to a particular level is based on performance rather than on academic preparation.
3. Evaluation is based on the job description and includes qualitative and quantitative factors.
4. Wages increase with each clinical level.

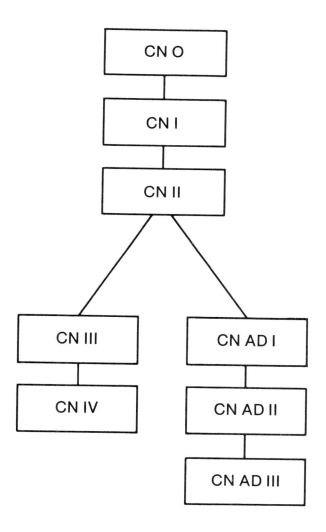

QUALIFICATIONS AND JOB SUMMARIES

Clinical Nurse Orientee	Clinical Nurse I	Clinical Nurse II	Clinical Nurse III	Clinical Nurse IV
JOB QUALIFICATIONS				
IP or registered nurse or R.N. returning to profession after prolonged absence or *may be* R.N. who has changed from one area of specialization to another.	Registered nurse or I.P. or R.N. returning to profession after prolonged absence or *is* R.N. who has changed from one area of specialization to another.	An experienced R.N. who has demonstrated ability to function as a CNII.	BS degree preferred. An experienced R.N. who has demonstrated ability to function as a C.N. III. Continues to fulfill C.N. II criteria.	An experienced R.N. who has demonstrated clinical expertise. M.S. degree in nursing required. (Placement at this level is subject to position available.)
DEGREE OF SUPERVISION				
1. Requires *direct close* supervision in a specific area of assignment for purposes of orientation *and/or during a* probationary period, in a controlled patient care situation. Gains knowledge and experience in initial application of policies.	1. Requires general supervision in specific area of assignment for purposes of orientation or specific assignment *following* probation in a controlled patient care situation. Incorporates policies into practice.	1. Works with *minimal* supervision. Promotes compliance in support of policies.	1. Works more independently with minimal supervision.	1. Works independently with collaborative supervision.

COMPLEXITY OF TASK

2. Performs routine patient care activities.

2. Performs routine patient care activities. Deals easily and successfully with common problems.

2. Demonstrates advanced clinical and communication skills. Solves complex clinical problems.

2. Demonstrates advanced clinical problem-solving and communication skills.

SCOPE OF PRACTICE

3. Performs established nursing procedures for individuals or *limited groups* of patients.

3. Performs established nursing procedures for individuals or groups of patients. Provides direct supervision to other members of the nursing team as assigned.

3. Identifies and implements nursing interventions and evaluates results of nursing interventions for a *given patient population.* Provides direct supervision/acts as resource to other members of the nursing team as assigned.

3. Recognized as having a specialty area of expertise. Functions as a resource in area expertise/coaches C.N.O., C.N. I, C.N. II and students. Participates in setting standards of care. Provides clinical staff development activities.

3. Assumes 24-hour responsibility as clinical resource/consultant for specialty area. Provides highly skilled and specialized direct/indirect patient care. Provides clinical staff development activities.

DEMONSTRATION OF PROFESSIONAL GROWTH

4. Establishes and expands personal clinical base of nursing knowledge and skills.

4. Continues to establish and expand personal clinical base of nursing knowledge and skills.

4. Functions as a professional role model. Achieves trust in professional colleagial relationships.

4. Is a leader in clinical practice. Demonstrates constructive/supportive approach in colleagial relationships.

4. Initiates and participates in nursing research. Collaborates with administrative nurses in:
   a) Developing

Clinical Nurse Orientee	Clinical Nurse I	Clinical Nurse II	Clinical Nurse III	Clinical Nurse IV
				quality assurance activities, b) initiating changes in nursing practice standard.

ORGANIZATIONAL RELATIONSHIPS

Clinical Nurse Orientee	Clinical Nurse I	Clinical Nurse II	Clinical Nurse III	Clinical Nurse IV
Accountable to: CN Ad I, CN Ad II	CN Ad I, CN Ad II	CN Ad I, CN Ad II	CN Ad I, CN Ad II	CN Ad II, CN Ad III, CN Ad IV

JOB QUALIFICATIONS IN PROGRESS FOR CN Ad I and CN Ad II.

LOMA LINDA UNIVERSITY MEDICAL CENTER

JOB DESCRIPTION

DIVISION: NURSING

JOB TITLE: CLINICAL NURSE SERIES — CN I and II

Effective 4/82 (Replaces 9/80)

GENERAL ENTRY LEVEL POSITION QUALIFICATIONS:

1. Current California nurse registration (or permittee [IP] status).
2. Knowledge/Skills/Commitment

   a. Ability to relate and work effectively with others.
   b. Demonstrated skills in verbal and written English communications for safe and effective patient care and to meet recording standards.
   c. Desire and potential for growth in skills and knowledge related to practice.
   d. Commitment to support Seventh-day Adventist health care philosophy.
   e. Willingness to comply with LLUMC Nursing Division and Departmental policies.
   f. Willingness to participate in goal-setting and educational activities for own professional advancement.

LLUMC CLINICAL NURSE LADDER

TITLE	JOB QUALIFICATIONS	POSITION SUMMARIES
Clinical Nurse Orientee (CNO)	Registered Nurse or IP or RN returning to profession after prolonged absence; or may be RN who has changed from one area of specialization to another.	Requires direct close supervision in specific area of assignment for purposes of orientation and/or during a probationary period, in a controlled patient care situation. Gains knowledge and experience in initial application of policies. Performs routine patient care activities. Performs established nursing procedures for individuals or limited groups of patients. Establishes and expands personal clinical base of nursing knowledge and skills.
Clinical Nurse I (CNI)	Registered Nurse (experience varies) or IP or RN who has changed from one area of specialization to another. This level begins after successful completion of the probationary period.	Requires general supervision in a controlled patient care situation. Incorporates policies into practice. Performs routine patient care activities. Deals easily and successfully with common problems. Performs established nursing procedures for individuals or groups of patients. Provides direct supervision to other members of the nursing team as assigned. Continues to establish and expand personal clinical base of nursing knowledge and skills.
Clinical Nurse II (CNII)	Experienced RN who has demonstrated ability to function as a CNII.	Works with minimal supervision. Promotes compliance and support of policies. Works with less predictable patient care situations. Identifies and implements nursing interventions for a given patient population. Provides direct supervision/acts as resource to other members of the nursing team as assigned. Functions as professional role model. Achieves trust in professional colleagial relationships.
Clinical Nurse III (CNIII)	BS degree preferred. Experienced RN who has demonstrated ability to function as a CNIII; continues to fulfill CNII criteria.	Works more independently with minimal supervision. Demonstrates advanced clinical and communication skills. Possesses a specialty area of expertise. Solves complex clinical problems. Provides clinical staff development activities. Functions as a resource in area of expertise/coaches CNO, CNI, CNII, and students. Participates in setting standards of care, and in developing policies and techniques. Is a leader in clinical practice. Demonstrates constructive/supportive approach in professional colleagial relationships.
Clinical Nurse IV (CNIV)	MS degree in Nursing. Experienced RN who has demonstrated clinical expertise. (Placement at this level is subject to position available.)	Works independently with/collaborative supervision. Assumes 24-hour responsibility as clinical resource/consultant for specialty area. Demonstrates advanced clinical problem-solving and communication skills. Provides highly skilled and specialized direct/indirect patient care. Initiates and participates in nursing research. Provides staff development activities. Collaborates with administrative nurses in: a. developing quality assurance activities. b. initiating changes in nursing practice standards.

LOMA LINDA UNIVERSITY MEDICAL CENTER
NURSING DIVISION

NURSE PRACTICE EXPECTATIONS AND EVALUATION
CLINICAL NURSE I AND II SERIES

Employee's Name		Title of present position		Unit	Shift

Hire Date	Length of time at present classification		Anniversary Date	
	Yrs	Mos		

Type of Evaluation	Period covered by this evaluation
□ Probationary □ Annual □ Interim □ Other _____	From _____ To _____ Mo _____ Day _____ Yr _____ Mo _____ Day _____ Yr _____

Evaluator's Signature	Title	Evaluation Date

At Loma Linda University Medical Center, the level of nursing can be determined by assessing the scope and depth of performance at which the nurse meets the established practice expectations.

The following are the beginning performance expectations for registered nurses at each level and their corresponding behavior evaluation. (Boxes blocked out indicate performance not required at that level):

A. CLINICAL COMPONENT

STANDARD I NURSING PROCESS

CNO	CNI	CNII	Develops, interprets and implements a plan of care for each patient through the nursing process:
□	□	□	• Obtains initial nursing history from patient or significant other
□	□	□	• Obtains ongoing patient history
□	□	□	• Acts appropriately on gathered information or observation — follows through
□	□	□	• Formulates and keeps care plans current with client input, giving evidence of knowledge of scientific and legal principles
□	□	□	• Implements a documented plan that reflects ongoing evaluation and collaboration with the total health team (including planning for next level of care)
□	□	□	• Documents care given according to LLUMC charting standards
□	□	□	• Facilitates patient's goals for physical, emotional and spiritual needs/comforts

COMMENTS: _____

_____

_____

_____

CNO: Identifies obvious patient problems based on limited job knowledge/skills with direct close supervision.
CNI: Identifies routine patient problems based on expanded job knowledge/skills with general supervision.
CNII: Requires minimal supervision except with complex situations. Reflects current nursing problem solving and takes responsibility for initiating change and utilizing resource people.

STANDARD II SAFETY/ENVIRONMENTAL CONTROL

CNO	CNI	CNII	Acts as advocate in providing safe delivery of care to promote wholeness.
□	■	■	• Receives passing grade on medication test
□	■	■	• Completes requirements for IV maintenance
			• Manages prescribed care of:
□	□	□	medications, IV's
□	□	□	procedures and techniques
			• Provides a safe environment by:
□	□	□	maintaining own physical health and mental alertness
□	□	□	managing and operating equipment securely
□	□	□	utilizing measures to prevent infection
□	□	□	responding calmly and effectively to emergency situations

COMMENTS: _____

_____

_____

CNO: Requires direct close supervision and guidance.
CNI: Works with general supervision in controlled situations. Is successful in routine situations, may need guidance in less predictable situations.
CNII: Successful in less predictable, more complex situations. Works with minimal supervision, identifying relationships and need for change. Able to evaluate results of care. Practice serve as professional role model/teacher.

35-0561 rev. (4-82) replaces (9-80)

STANDARD III PROFESSIONAL RESPONSIBILITIES

Needs Improvement	Yes	
☐	☐	Fulfills professional responsibility to the institution in adherence to philosophy and general policy.
☐	☐	• Fulfills attendance requirements
☐	☐	• Adheres to dress code
☐	☐	• Accepts reasonable assignment (on or off unit)
☐	☐	• Maintains current C.P.R. certification
☐	☐	• Attends required hospital safety programs

COMMENTS: _____

OTHER CERTIFICATIONS: _____

B. EDUCATION COMPONENT
STANDARD IV EDUCATION

Imparts knowledge to meet needs on a one-to-one or group basis either formally or informally (this includes teaching and instructing in order to facilitate reaching short and long range goals).

CNO	CNI	CNII	Patients, families, significant others
■	☐	☐	• Anticipates patient learning needs for changing levels of care including preparation for discharge
☐	☐	☐	• Initiates appropriate teaching
☐	☐	☐	• Documents teaching related activities and response to information given
■	☐	☐	• Identifies further teaching needs based on response to previous instruction
☐	☐	☐	• Utilizes resource persons as indicated

COMMENTS: _____

CNO: Demonstrates skills and intered in learing by observation and supervised participation.
CNI: Provides routine teaching with general superivision, seeks assistance for more complex teaching needs.
CNII: Skilled in complex and unusual teaching; teaching demonstrates advanced assessment skills and creativity. Serves as a role model to staff and patients.

CNO	CNI	CNII	Staff
■	☐	☐	• Demonstrates initiative in the orientation of new staff
☐	☐	☐	• Facilitates staff attendance of programs and conferences
☐	☐	☐	• Shows concern for staff growth by participation in teaching sessions, team conferences
☐	☐	☐	• Demonstrates openness to instruction and guidance
☐	☐	☐	• Looks for learning opportunities

COMMENTS: _____

CNO: Shares with and learns from peer group in expanding nursing and knowledge skills.
CNI: Provides routine teaching with general supervision, seeks assistance for more complex teaching needs.
CNII: Skilled in complex and unusual teaching; teaching demonstrates advanced assessment skills and creativity. Serve as a role model to staff and patients.

CNO	CNI	CNII	Students
■	☐	☐	• Provides teaching for students by involving them in unit activities that will enchance their learning
■	☐	☐	• Functions as professional role model
☐	☐	☐	• Communicates with instructor regarding performance

COMMENTS: _____

CNO: Receptive to students' needs.
CNI: Provides accurate information in routine situations and involves resource persons in more complex situations.
CNII: Assists in teaching students in less predictable patient care situations. Practice serves as a role model.

STANDARD V PROFESSIONAL GROWTH

No	Yes	Practice reflects current developments in the profession.
☐	☐	• Participates in educational programs related to areas of practice
☐	☐	• Aids in expanding/validating the basis of nursing practice (i.e., research)

COMMENTS: _____

_____
_____
_____
_____

Expected at all levels

C. MANAGEMENT COMPONENT
STANDARD VI PROFESSIONAL MANAGEMENT

CNO	CNI	CNII	Demonstrates personal attributes and behaviors which enhance management and clinical practice.
☐	☐	☐	• Delegates reasonable assignment impartially
☐	☐	☐	• Sets Priorities
☐	☐	☐	• Utilizes times efficiently
☐	☐	☐	• Demonstrates insight in decision making
☐	☐	☐	• Demonstrates effectual problem solving
☐	☐	☐	• Practices self direction
☐	☐	☐	• Interrelates productively/tactfully with:
☐	☐	☐	peers
☐	☐	☐	staff
☐	☐	☐	medical staff
☐	☐	☐	other departments
☐	☐	☐	patients
☐	☐	☐	families
☐	☐	☐	• Manifests positive behavior change in response to instruction and guidance

COMMENTS: _____

_____
_____
_____

CNO: Requires direct, close supervision.
CNI: Requires general supervision.
CNII: Works with minimal supervision and utilizes resources.

SUMMARY: _____

_____

_____

_____

_____

_____

_____

_____

_____

_____

_____

_____

_____

_____

_____

_____

I have reviewed the foregoing evaluation. I understand the goals mutually agreed upon and their significance as related to my future performance.

_____

_____

_____

_____

_____

_____

_____

_____

_____

_____

_____

_____

_____

Employee _____ Date _____

Evaluator _____
                              RN

Mary Greeley Medical Center

Ames, Iowa

217 Beds

Performance Evaluation Forms:
  Licensed Practical Nurse
  Patient Care Coordinator
  Nurse Manager
Nursing Diagnosis Module
  Nursing Diagnosis Pretest
  Nursing Diagnosis Work Sheet #1
  Nursing Diagnosis Work Sheet #2
  Nursing Diagnosis Work Sheet #3

Reprinted by permission of Phyllis Crouse, Assistant Administrator, Director of Nursing

MARY GREELEY MEDICAL CENTER
Ames, Iowa

Nursing Department
PERFORMANCE EVALUATION

Name: _____   Classification: Licensed Practical Nurse

Nursing Unit: _____   Period of Evaluation: _____

Rating: 4 points - Exceeds Standards (Performs at this level 90%+ of time)
         2 points - Meets Standards (Performs at this level 75-89% of time)
         0 points - Does Not Meet Standards (Performs below 75% of time)

FACTORS (From Performance Standards)	WEIGHT	Rating 4 ,2 ,0	POINTS	COMMENTS
A. Clinical Practice				
Nursing Activity	60%			
1. Interviews patients ...	(10)			
2. Performs designated ...	(10)			
3. Seeks guidance ...	(10)			
7. Observes symptoms ...	(10)			
8. Acts to maintain ...	(10)			
9. Assists the R.N. ...	(10)			
Accountability	10%			
4. Attends conferences ...	(5)			
5. Takes appropriate action...	(5)			
Communication	5%			
6. Communicates clearly ...				
10. Assists in patient ed. ...				
11. Participates in ...				
B. Administration	10%			
C. Education/Personal Development	10%			
D. Research	5%			

TOTAL   100%

Developmental needs, goals, strong points, and additional comments:

_____
_____
_____
_____
_____
_____
_____
_____
_____
_____
_____
_____

                              Reviewed (initial)

_____ _____ _____
Evaluator's Signature & Title, Date Dept. Head, Date Ass't. Adm., Date

Employee's Comments: _____
_____
_____
_____
_____
_____
_____
_____

                              Reviewed (initial)

_____ _____ _____
Employee's Signature, Date   Dept. Head, Date Ass't. Adm., Date

MARY GREELEY MEDICAL CENTER
Ames, Iowa

Nursing Department
PERFORMANCE EVALUATION

Name: _____   Classification: <u>Patient Care Coordinator</u>

Nursing Unit: _____   Period of Evaluation: _____

Rating: 4 points - Exceeds Standards (Performs at this level 90%+ of time)
2 points - Meets Standards (Performs at this level 75-89% of time)
0 points - Does Not Meet Standards (Performs below 75% of time)

FACTORS (From Performance Standards)	WEIGHT	Rating 4 2 0	POINTS	COMMENTS
I. To the Assist. Administrator/ Director of Nursing	45%			
A. Organizational 10%				
B. Operational 15%				
C. Communications 15%				
D. Developmental 5%				
II. To Divisional Personnel	25%			
A. Operational 10%				
B. Orientation 5%				
C. Communications 5%				
D. Developmental 5%				
III. To Medical Staff	10%			
A. Operational 5%				
B. Communications 5%				
IV. To Other Departments	10%			
A. Operational 5%				
B. Communications 5%				
V. To Other Organizations	5%			
A. Communications				
B. Developmental				
VI. To Self	5%			
A. Developmental				

TOTAL   <u>100%</u>

Developmental needs, goals, strong points, and additional comments:

_____
_____
_____
_____
_____
_____
_____
_____
_____
_____
_____
_____

Reviewed (initial)

Evaluator's Signature & Title, Date   Dept. Head, Date   Ass't. Adm., Date

Employee's Comments: _____

_____
_____
_____
_____
_____
_____
_____

Reviewed (initial)

Employee's Signature, Date   Dept. Head, Date   Ass't. Adm., Date

MARY GREELEY MEDICAL CENTER
Ames, Iowa

Nursing Department
PERFORMANCE EVALUATION

Name: _____   Classification: ___Nurse Manager___

Nursing Unit: _____   Period of Evaluation: _____

Rating: 4 points - Exceeds Standards (Performs at this level 90%+ of time)
          2 points - Meets Standards (Performs at this level 75-89% of time)
          0 points - Does Not Meet Standards (Performs below 75% of time)

FACTORS (From Performance Standards)	WEIGHT	Rating 4 2 0	POINTS	COMMENTS
A. To Patient/Significant Other	30%			
B. To Medical Staff	10%			
C. To Other Staff	30%			
D. To Nursing Administration	20%			
E. To Other Department Personnel	5%			
F. To Self	5%			

TOTAL   100%

Developmental needs, goals, strong points, and additional comments:

_____
_____
_____
_____
_____
_____
_____
_____
_____
_____
_____
_____

Reviewed (initial)

Evaluator's Signature & Title, Date   Dept. Head, Date   Ass't. Adm., Date

Employee's Comments: _____

_____
_____
_____
_____
_____
_____
_____

Reviewed (initial)

Employee's Signature, Date   Dept. Head, Date   Ass't. Adm., Date

MARY GREELEY MEDICAL CENTER
Ames, Iowa

Nursing Education Department

NURSING DIAGNOSIS SELF-LEARNING MODULE FOR
R.N. CLINICAL LADDER*

Upon completion of this module the nurse will be able to make a nursing diagnosis and formulate nursing interventions specific to the individual patient. The objectives are as follows:

1. Will be able to identify and write an acceptable nursing diagnosis utilizing the nursing process.
2. Demonstrates ability to differentiate nursing diagnosis from medical diagnosis.
3. Documents the nursing diagnosis on the patient care plan.
4. Documentation in the medical records reflects the nursing diagnosis and related nursing interventions.

Directions:

1. Obtain the pretest from Nursing Education.
2. Upon completion of the pretest, obtain from Nursing Education the following:
   a. List of required readings.
   b. Work Sheets #1, #2 and #3.
   Nursing Education will review work completed on the work sheets. If unsatisfactory performance is noted, the learner will be asked to repeat the work sheets.
3. Over a three-month (90-day) period of time, 80 percent of charts audited by the Nurse Manager will reflect documentation of the nursing diagnosis on the nursing care plan and in the nurse's notes. This three-month (90-day) time period will start at the indication of the learner after she/he has completed the pretest and required readings and feels comfortable writing nursing diagnoses. The actual number of charts audited will be up to the individual Nurse Manager

---

* Developed by Fran Venter, R.N., Nursing Education Department, with contributors Mary Carr, R.N., N.M., 2 East; Marilyn Polito, R.N., N.M., E.D.; and Linda Vogtlin, R.N., H.M.

but must be able to accurately reflect the learner's ability to make a nursing diagnosis (i.e., 8 out of 10 charts, 12 out of 15 charts, etc.).

4. Following completion of the above, a posttest will be given. A passing grade of 80 percent must be attained for satisfactory completion of this module.

MARY GREELEY MEDICAL CENTER
Ames, Iowa

Nursing Education Department

NURSING DIAGNOSIS MODULE

Content:

☐ Pretest
☐ Required Readings

    ☐ "Nursing Diagnosis," Chapter 8 in *Nursing Process: Application of Theories, Frameworks and Models* by Janet W. Griffith and Paula J. Christensen.
    ☐ "Nursing Diagnosis," *Nursing 81*, June 1981, p. 34.
    ☐ "What's Your Diagnosis," *RN*, October 1980, p. 63.
    ☐ Nursing Diagnosis: "Making a Concept Come Alive," *AJN*, April 1980, p. 668.
    ☐ "The Nursing Process and Maslow's Human Need Theory," Chapter 3 in *Nursing Diagnosis and Intervention in Nursing Practice*, by Claire Campbell.
    ☐ "The Impact of Nursing Diagnosis," *AORN*, May 1975. (copy available from Nursing Education)

☐ Work Sheets
    ☐ Work Sheet # 1—Differentiating Between Nursing and Medical Diagnoses
    ☐ Work Sheet # 2—Case Study: Writing Nursing Diagnoses
    ☐ Work Sheet # 3—Case Study: Incorporating Nursing Diagnoses Into Your Care Plan

☐ Clinical Application
  ☐ 80% of charts reflect documentation of the nursing diagnosis on the
    care plan and in the nurse's notes over a 3-month (90-day) period.
        Signed _____, Nurse Manager

☐ Posttest—Has successfully completed posttest with a score of 80% or
  above.
        Signed _____, Nursing Ed. Coordinator

☐ Successful completion of Nursing Diagnosis Module.

New 3/83 Fran Venter, R.N./mt

MARY GREELEY MEDICAL CENTER
Ames, Iowa

Nursing Education Department

NURSING DIAGNOSIS PRETEST

1. Define nursing diagnosis.

2. How is a nursing diagnosis different from a patient problem?

3. Explain how a nursing diagnosis fits into the nursing process.

4. Describe the differences between nursing diagnosis and medical diagnosis.

5. Explain the difference between needs and problems.

6. Write two nursing diagnostic statements using this case:

   You are taking care of a 34-year-old male who is complaining of severe right-sided chest pain. The chest x-ray shows slight infiltrate in the right upper lobe which is suggestive of either a pneumonia or pulmonary embolus. The vital signs are as follows: temperature 99.2 (oral), pulse 110, respirations 28 and shallow. Skin cool and clammy. Patient is verbalizing fears about dying. Wife is at bedside crying softly and expressing fears about money problems should the patient die.

   1.

   2.

7. List four steps involved in arriving at a diagnostic statement.

   1.

   2.

   3.

   4.

8. List three reasons for keeping nursing diagnoses updated.

   1.

   2.

   3.

9. Who determines which nursing diagnoses are acceptable?

10. Define a nursing order and describe its relation to the nursing diagnosis.

New 3/83 Fran Venter, R.N./mt

NURSING DIAGNOSIS WORK SHEET # 1

Differentiating Between Nursing and Medical Diagnoses

Please read each statement and determine if it is a nursing diagnosis or a medical diagnosis. For each medical diagnosis, rewrite in a nursing diagnosis format.

1. Anxiety related to upcoming mastectomy.

2. Altered ability to perform self-care activities related to fractured wrist.

3. Cold fingers related to brachial emboli.

4. Pulmonary emboli related to increased clotting of blood.

5. Potential overload of body fluids related to low urine output.

6. Understanding deficit related to unfamiliarity with illness, treatment, and diagnostic procedures.

7. Hypoglycemia related to diabetes.

8. Communication impairment related to tracheostomy.

9. Confusion related to lost hearing aid.

10. Depression related to loss of right breast.

11. Broken hip related to fall from bed.

12. Circulation impairment related to prolonged bed rest.

13. Alterations in nutrition related to nasogastric tube.

14. Impairment of bowel function related to recent ileostomy.

15. Pulmonary edema related to renal failure.

16. Ear drainage related to head injury.

17. Sleep deprivation related to necessity for frequent vital signs.

18. Vaginal bleeding related to imminent miscarriage.

19. Pain related to dressing changes.

20. Impairment of cough effort related to thoracotomy incision.

21. Cold toes related to blocked popliteal artery.

22. Potential for impairment of skin integrity related to prolonged bed rest.

23. Swollen hand related to fractured wrist.

24. Alteration in comfort level related to hip spica cast.

25. Confusion related to organic brain syndrome.

New 3/83 Fran Venter, R.N./mt

NURSING DIAGNOSIS WORK SHEET # 2

Case Study: Writing Nursing Diagnoses

Read through the following case studies and write three nursing diagnostic statements for each:

Case # 1

> Mrs. B, a 38-year-old female, is admitted to the Short Stay Unit of Mary Greeley Medical Center in preparation for a tubal fulguration. The nurse in charge of Mrs. B does the preoperative teaching and begins to prep the lower abdomen. Mrs. B becomes upset when she sees the nurse is about to shave some of her pubic hair. "I don't think this is necessary!" she says and pulls her gown down. After some explanation, the nurse helps Mrs. B to realize the importance of removal of the pubic hair in regard to her surgery.
>
> Thirty minutes later Mrs. B tells the nurse that she has had two loose stools due to her nervousness. The nurse questions Mrs. B further and finds out Mrs. B has a fear that she will not wake up from her anesthetic. The nurse reassures Mrs. B about the anesthesia used and offers to call the Anesthesiologist in so he can answer any questions Mrs. B may have. Mrs. B refuses, stating "I'm sure everything will be fine" while looking down at her sheets.
>
> Ten minutes before Mrs. B's scheduled surgical procedure the charge nurse receives a phone call from the surgeon's nurse, who informs the charge nurse that two C-sections will be done before Mrs. B's tubal fulguration. When the nurse tells Mrs. B her surgery will be delayed approximately two hours, Mrs. B starts crying and states, "He promised me he'd do it right at 8 o'clock! I can't wait any longer!"

Note: Cases #2 through #5 for work sheet #2 have been omitted.

NURSING DIAGNOSIS WORK SHEET # 3

Incorporating Nursing Diagnoses Into Your Care Plan

Read through the following case studies and write three nursing diagnostic statements for each. Then write a care plan for each case study utilizing the three nursing diagnostic statements you have formulated. Show how your nursing diagnosis fits into the nursing process.

Case Study # 1

Mr. T. J. is a 50-year-old male being admitted to your nursing unit for an elective right herniorrhaphy.

I. History of Presenting Problem

Patient discovered the hernia himself 3½ months ago. He is able to reduce it himself and finds he must do so 2–3 times a day. He considers this to be a nuisance and an inconvenience. There is no pain involved but activities are somewhat restricted now. The patient is concerned that he will not be able to keep up with work and hobbies if he does not have this surgery. Apprehensive about surgery. Was actually scheduled six weeks ago but patient postponed it. States he just was not sure he wanted it done.

II. Physical and Sensory Data

Loose productive cough evident. Patient attributes this to too much smoking. 2–2½ packs/day for past 20 years. Small reddened crusty patches noted on both elbows and around hairline. Patient states this is psoriasis. Otherwise skin intact— color good.

Patient is nearsighted. Wears glasses all the time. Hearing is good. Mouth is well hydrated, teeth in good dental repair. No dentures or removable bridges.

Usually has B.M. daily. Occasional constipation when travelling. No difficulty voiding. Usually gets up once during the night to void.

Below-the-knee amputation on right leg due to injury at work 15 years ago. Uses leg prosthesis very well. Is able to apply and remove prosthesis himself.

BP 154/96
TPR 98^8 - 72 - 16 (AP regular)
Ht 6'2" Wt 205
Skin warm and dry—good color

III. Personal Habits and Social Data

Sleeps 6–8 hours nightly. Usually retires around 11 PM after showering. Eats three meals a day. Very little snacking—just

III. *Personal Habits and Social Data* (continued)

popcorn once a week or so. Tries to watch cholesterol by not eating too many eggs—average 3/week. Does not drink. Has never tried mood-altering (street) drugs.

Lives with wife and two sons. Eighteen-year-old son is about to graduate from high school. Twenty-two-year-old son is in college but lives at home. Twenty-six-year-old daughter is married and lives in St. Louis.

Hobbies include gardening, fishing, and reading. Occupation is maintenance supervisor at John Deere. Has worked there 21 years and enjoys his work. He uses an electric scooter at work so he does not have to do a lot of walking.

IV. *Medical History*

Has had hypertension for 1½ years. Has been taking diuril for this. Patient is quite concerned about hypertension because father and brother died from strokes.

Allergic to Ampicillin (gets a skin rash) and ragweed (sneezing and swollen eyes)

Meds—One-a-day vitamins—takes daily. Last dose this AM.
        Diuril 500mg bid—last dose this AM.
        Allerest—prn late Summer and Fall only—last dose in November.

Familial history of hypertension and strokes. No history of diabetes.

Previous hospitalizations include:
    1949—Appendectomy
    1963—Right leg (below the knee) amputation
    1964—Stump revision
    1976—Diagnosis and treatment of hypertension

Note: Other case studies have been omitted.

BIBLIOGRAPHY

Campbell, Claire. *Nursing Diagnosis and Intervention in Nursing Practice.* New York: John Wiley & Sons, Inc., 1978, Chapter 3.

Christensen, Paula J., and Griffith, Janet W. *Nursing Process: Application of Theories, Frameworks and Model.* St. Louis: The C.V. Mosby Company, 1982, Chapter 8.

del Bueno, Dorothy, et al. "What's Your Diagnosis?" *RN,* October 1980, pp. 63–106.

Disbrow, Mildred, et al. *Maternity Nursing Case Studies*. Medical Examination Publishing Co., Inc., 1976, p. 91.

Dossey, Barbara, and Guzzetta, Cathie E. "Nursing Diagnosis." *Nursing 81*, June 1981, *30*(6), pp. 34–38.

Johnson, Mae M., and Davis, Mary Lou C. *Problem Solving in Nursing Practice*. Dubuque, Iowa: William C. Brown Company, Publishers, 1975, p. 121.

Price, Mary Radatovich. "Making a Concept Come Alive." *American Journal of Nursing,* April 1980, *80*(4), pp. 668–671.

Roy, Sister Callista. "The Impact of Nursing Diagnosis." *AORN Journal,* May 1975, pp. 1023–1030.

Wooley, F. Ross, et al. *Problem-Oriented Nursing*. New York: Springer Publishing Co., Inc., 1974.

Appendix G 267

The Moses H. Cone Memorial Hospital

Greensboro, N.C.

456 Beds

IN APPRECIATION

The Clinical Career Tracks Task Force expresses its appreciation to the nursing staff at Evanston Hospital, Evanston, Illinois and to Porter Memorial Hospital, Denver, Colorado for sharing their career track programs with us. We truly benefited from their pioneering efforts and were able to cut months of preparation time from our implementation schedule. A special thanks to Joanne Pervorse of Porter Memorial Hospital for her support and help during our initial planning stages.

ACKNOWLEDGEMENT

The Chairman of the Clinical Career Tracks Task Force wishes to acknowledge the countless hours and hard work of the following persons toward the establishment of this program:

Susan Bays, RN, MSN	Instructor, Staff Development
Betty Bauguess, RN	Head Nurse, Coronary Care Unit
LaVonne Beach, RN, MSN	Head Nurse, Post-partum Unit
Sue Booth, RN	Asst. Head Nurse, Emergency Room
Terri Burleson, RN, BSN	Asst. Head Nurse, Labor & Delivery
Kim Cates, RN, BSN	Staff Nurse, Pediatrics
Candy Colglazier, RN, BSN	Nursing Consultant
Ethel Hall, RN, MSN	Nursing Consultant
Cathy Hamlin, RN, BSN	Asst. Head Nurse, Psychiatry
Myrtle Hardin, RN, BSN	Asst. Head Nurse, Medical
Susan Harvey, RN, MSN	Nursing Consultant
Rebecca Jenkins, RN	Staff Nurse, Orthopedics
Cynthia Marcum, RN	Staff Nurse, Nursery
Linda McNeal, RN, MSN	Staff Nurse, MICU
Faye Oliver, RN	Staff Nurse, Surgery
Jo Anne Rayle, RN, MSN	Instructor, Staff Development
Linda Roberts, RN, MSN	Clinical Specialist, Medical
Cheryl Royal, RN, BSN	Head Nurse, SICU
Peggy Shoffner, RN	Staff Nurse, Medical
Naomi Stewart, RN, BSN	Asst. Head Nurse, Progressive Care
Jane Schrock, RN	Staff Nurse, Surgical
Kathy Utz, RN, BSN	Staff Nurse, Labor & Delivery

Ann M. Fonville, RN, MPH Chairman

Note: Sections III and IV of the program manual are omitted due to space limitations.

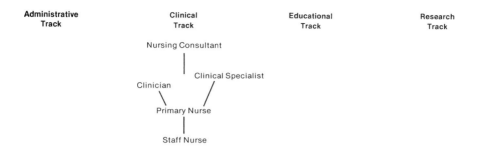

SECTION I: INTRODUCTION AND PHILOSOPHY

A. Introduction to Levels of Clinical Practice: Purpose and Objectives

The purposes of the Clinical Career Track of the Department of Nursing are to provide recognition for excellence in nursing practice and to promote the advancement of professional nursing.

This will be accomplished by adherence to the departmental philosophy and by the dedication of administrators and educators in supporting nurses in clinical practice.

The Department of Nursing provides the process and opportunities that will:

1. Encourage the nurse to plan career goals, direct efforts to meet performance criteria, and apply for positions to meet the career goals.
2. Enable the nurse to move upward or laterally as the individual is able to meet the performance criteria for available positions.
3. Support the upward mobility of the nurse by a planned salary scale that provides increased financial remuneration as clinical competence and responsibility increase.

Note: Six pages of narrative descriptions of the clinical career tracks have been omitted.

The Moses H. Cone Memorial Hospital Department of Nursing Clinical Career Progression Table

	Staff Nurse	Primary Nurse	Clinician	Clinical Specialist
Education	Current North Carolina license to practice nursing.	Current North Carolina license to practice nursing.	Current North Carolina license to practice nursing. Baccalaureate degree in health-related field* and evidence of advanced study and/or certification in field.	Current North Carolina license to practice nursing. Master's in Nursing is required and certification in field (if available) recommended within two (2) years of appointment.
Experience	No previous experience required.	Satisfactory performance at Staff Nurse level or one to two years' recent experience acute care setting.	Minimum of four (4) years' experience in acute care setting; at least three (3) years in clinical specialty	Minimum of four (4) years in acute care setting; at least three (3) years in clinical specialty.
Clinical Knowledge	Demonstrates ability to function at Level I job description and skills list (Required Competencies). Demonstrates understanding of basic principles and policies of professional nursing	Demonstrates ability to function at Level II job description and skills list prior to promotion to this position within three months of employment. Demonstrates evidence of principles	Demonstrates ability to function at Level III job description and skills list prior to promotion to this position or within three months of employment. Demonstrates broad knowledge in clinical	Demonstrates in-depth, advanced knowledge of the current professional nursing theory, practice, and techniques in area of specialty. Effectively utilizes the nursing process.

* For registered nurses employed before April 1, 1982, ten (10) years of experience will be accepted in lieu of a Baccalaureate degree. This option expires January 1, 1983.

using the nursing process.	and practice of professional nursing and practical application of knowledge in clinical area using the nursing process.	specialty area applying the nursing process.	Demonstrates ability to function at Level IV job description and skills list prior to promotion to this position or within three months of employment. Demonstrates broad knowledge in clinical specialty area applying the nursing process.
Hospital Affiliations	Serves on Unit Committees as assigned or by individual's request.	Serves on unit and intradepartment committees and task forces as assigned or by individual's request.	Serves on unit, department-mental, or hospital committees or task forces as assigned or by individual's request.	Serves on unit, department-mental, or hospital committees and task forces as assigned or by individual's request.
Professional Affiliations	Involvement in professional and community activities is supported and encouraged.	Involvement in professional and community activities is supported and encouraged.	Involvement in professional and community activities is supported and encouraged.	Involvement in professional and community activities is supported and encouraged.
Certification	Attains certification as Basic Rescuer in CPR within three months of	Currently certified as Basic Rescuer in CPR.	Currently certified as Instructor in CPR and teaches at least one	Currently certified as Instructor in CPR and teaches at least one

	Staff Nurse	Primary Nurse	Clinician	Clinical Specialist
	employment and maintains yearly recertification.		(1) hospital-based class/year.	(1) hospital-based class/year.
Continuing Education	Attends at least twenty (20) hours of continuing education per year. Attends at least 75 percent of scheduled unit meetings per year.	Attends at least thirty (30) hours of continuing education per year. Demonstrates evidence of change in nursing practice as a result of continuing education. Attends at least 75 percent of scheduled unit meetings.	Attends at least thirty (30) hours of continuing education per year, at least 15 hours of which are in area of clinical specialty. Demonstrates evidence of change in nursing practice as a result of continuing education. Attends at least 75 percent of scheduled unit meetings, conducts service-based education programs.	Attends at least thirty (30) hours of continuing education per year, at least 15 hours of which are in area of clinical specialty. Demonstrates evidence of change in nursing practice as a result of continuing education. Attends at least 75 percent of scheduled unit meetings, conducts service-based education programs.
Research	Participates in clinical research as requested.	Participates in clinical research as requested.	Assists in conducting clinical research in area of specialty.	Initiates and conducts clinical research in area of specialty.
Interpersonal Skills	Communicates with patients, families, students, and staff.	Is a positive role model. Establishes and maintains rapport	Is a positive role model. Exhibits leadership abilities. Estab-	Is a positive role model. Communicates effectively with

with patients, families, students, and staff. Exhibits beginning leadership skills.	lishes and maintains rapport with patients, families, students, and staff.	patients, families, students, and staff. Knowledgeable in problem solving, decision making, leadership, and group process skills.

SECTION II. CAREER PROGRESSION REVIEW COMMITTEE

A. Purpose:

The Career Progression Review Committee will review the candidates for *Level III, Clinician* and *Level IV, Clinical Specialist* positions and make a recommendation to the Head Nurse for or against promotion.

B. Policy:

1. The Career Progression Review Committee meets during the last month of each calendar quarter.
2. The committee is chaired by the Administrator/Assistant Administrator of Nursing. After the first year the chairmanship may rotate to an experienced committee member who has been through the Promotion Review process.
3. Committee members are appointed by the Administrator/Assistant Administrator of Nursing to serve two- (2)-year terms.
4. All terms begin in January and half of the committee is appointed every year.
5. Each clinical practice area has at least one (1) representative.
6. The Administrator/Assistant Administrator may appoint alternates to fill committee membership as needed. Care is taken to see that representation from all position levels and clinical practice areas is maintained.
7. No formal action of the committee is taken unless a minimum of seven (7) committee members are in attendance.
8. Each candidate is assigned a sponsor from the committee membership.

C. Composition:

1. The committee is composed of (the annual rotation pattern appears in parentheses):
   a. Assistant Administrator/Administrator
   b. Clinical Director (even year)
   c. Nursing Consultant (odd year)
   d. Head Nurse (even year)
   e. Assistant Head Nurse (odd year)
   f. Clinical Specialist (even year)
   g. Clinician (odd year)
   h. Staff Development Instructor (even year)

      i. Staff Nurse/Primary Nurse (odd year)
      j. Staff Nurse/Primary Nurse (even year)
      k. Staff Nurse/Primary Nurse (odd year)
  2. The chairman may appoint ad hoc nonvoting members for clinical expertise as needed.

D. Procedure:

1. The committee chairman schedules the committee to meet during the last month of each calendar quarter.
2. Career Progression Review files of all candidates are submitted to the committee chairman by the first month of the calendar quarter.
3. The committee chairman posts the following on all nursing units four (4) weeks prior to the committee review:
   a. Names of all candidates
   b. Clinical area
   c. Position sought
   d. Names of the committee members
   e. Procedure for Unsolicited Recommendations
4. All Unsolicited Recommendations must be individually signed and submitted to the committee chairman two (2) weeks prior to the committee review.
5. The committee chairman notifies the committee members of the review meeting date, time, and place.
6. All committee members review all candidates' files one (1) week prior to the scheduled meeting. Files are maintained in the Nursing Administration office to protect confidentiality.
7. The committee chairman notifies the candidates of the review meeting date, time, and place.
8. The committee chairman notifies all ad hoc members of meeting date, time, and place. The ad hoc members are provided the opportunity to review selected Career Progression Review candidate files in the Nursing Administration office.
9. Each appointed sponsor meets individually with his/her candidate prior to the committee review date to assist the candidate in preparing for the committee interview.
10. The sponsor introduces the candidate to the Review Committee members and supports the candidate throughout the review process.
11. The chairman conducts the Career Progression Review meeting and advises the members about the review process. The chairman emphasizes that all committee proceedings are confidential.

12. The committee interviews each candidate to ascertain the candidate's qualifications and goals for the position sought.
13. The committee submits to the Head Nurse a written recommendation for or against the promotion of each candidate. A copy of this report goes to the Clinical Director and a copy is sent to the candidate (at home address). *This report is treated as confidential!*
14. The contents of the Career Progression Review file, with the exception of the Peer Recommendations, are placed in the candidate's personal folder. A summary of all Peer Recommendations is made and added to the personnel folder. All Peer Recommendation data sheets are destroyed.

Schedule of Events

JAN/APR/JUL/OCT.	1. First month of each calendar quarter all candidates must be submitted to Committee Chairman.
FEB/MAY/AUG/ NOV.	1. Four weeks prior to Committee Meeting, Chairman posts all candidates' data on all nursing units.
	2. Two weeks prior to committee meeting, all Unsolicited Peer Recommendations are submitted to Committee Chairman.
	3. One week prior to committee meeting, all files are ready for review by committee members during that week.
MAR/JUN/SEP/ DEC.	1. Committee meets during the last month of each calendar quarter.

Note: Sections III and IV of manual—Career progression data sheets and procedure for withdrawal of application—have been omitted.

SECTION V: CAREER PROGRESSION POLICY AND PROCEDURE AND REQUIRED COMPETENCIES: CLINICAL TRACK

Level I—Staff Nurse

1. *Policy:*
   Staff Nurse is the entry level position intended for new graduates and registered nurses who have not had recent experience in an acute

care setting. After three (3) months of employment, the nurse who has demonstrated mastery of the Staff Nurse (Level I) job description and required competencies, *and* who has shown ability to function under the Primary Nurse (Level II) job description and required competencies, may apply to the Head Nurse for promotion. Promotion to Primary Nurse is subject to position availability.

2. *Procedure:*
   a. The candidate:
      1. applies for a Staff Nurse position by completing a routine hospital job application.
      2. is interviewed by the Nurse Recruiter, Clinical Director, and/ or Head Nurse.
   b. The Head Nurse meets with each new Staff Nurse and:
      1. explains the Staff Nurse job description and required competencies.
      2. outlines the procedure for promotion via the Clinical Career Progression Program.
   c. All Nurse Interns enter at Staff Nurse (Level I) and may apply for promotion at the conclusion of their internship.

PERFORMANCE EVALUATION

EMPLOYEE (NAME): _____ POSITION TITLE: **STAFF NURSE**
DEPARTMENT: _____ TIME IN POSITION: _____
SUPERVISOR (NAME): _____ EMPLOYMENT DATE: _____
SUPERVISOR (TITLE): _____

DATE OF LAST PERFORMANCE REVIEW: _____

Abbreviated Major Work Activities (Review the major work activities on the position description and use the key words to describe each area.) List major work activities in descending order of importance. Insert comments if performance is above or below Competent.

| | *Performance* | |
| *(P or S)** | *Rating* | *Comments* |

1. (P) Assesses patient needs.   _____
                                  _____
                                  _____

2. (P) Plans individualized care _____
        based on patient assess- _____
        ment and nursing his-   _____
        tory.   _____

3. (P) Implements the plan of   _____
        care according to estab- _____
        lished standards.   _____

4. (P) Evaluates pt. care based _____
        on pt. outcomes, analy-   _____
        sis of written data, and _____
        communication w/other   _____
        health care providers.   _____

5. (P) Communicates effec-   _____
        tively verbally and in   _____
        writing.   _____

6. (S) Follows established poli- _____
        cies and procedures.   _____
                                  _____

7. (S) Participates in unit com- _____
        mittees as appropriate.   _____
                                  _____

8. (S) Assists with clinical   _____
        research as requested.   _____
                                  _____

9. ( ) _____   _____
        _____   _____
        _____   _____

* Next to the major work activity ( ) indicate if you consider it to be "Primary" (P) or "Secondary" (S)

Primary (P)—Most important results areas. Position must accomplish primary work activities to be effective. These primary areas are "make-or-break" aspects of the job.

Secondary (S)—These accountabilities support accomplishment of primary work activities.

CLINICAL CAREER TRACK: LEVEL I—STAFF NURSE

Required Competencies

The Required Competencies for the Clinical Career Track identify the nursing knowledge and skills expected at each level. It is expected that the nurse at any level be able to demonstrate the required competencies for all preceding levels. *Prior to promotion the nurse must demonstrate the required competencies* for the position being sought.

Key: P & P—policy and procedure reference
Read P & P—has read policy and procedure
Demo Comp—has demonstrated competency
N.A.—not applicable or not available in particular clinical specialty

P & P	REQUIRED COMPETENCIES	READ P & P	DEMO COMP	N.A.	COMMENTS
		DATE & INITIAL EACH ENTRY			
	Level I—Staff Nurse				
	I. Assessment				
	A. Completes patient data base on admission to the Unit according to unit/service standards.				
	B. Utilizes effective interviewing skills to elicit pertinent information.				
	C. Assesses patient condition using inspection, palpation, ausculation, and percussion; appropriately communicates deviation(s) from normal.				
	D. Recognizes pathophysiology and incorporates in care plan.				
	E. Interprets diagnostic/monitoring data: 1. Recognizes significance based upon patient's condition.				
	2. Reports abnormal data.				
	3. Initiates appropriate intervention.				
	F. Accurately identifies nursing diagnoses for primary patients.				

P & P	REQUIRED COMPETENCIES	READ P & P	DEMO COMP	N.A.	COMMENTS
		DATE & INITIAL EACH ENTRY			
	Level I—Staff Nurse				
	G. Documents patient data and nursing diagnoses using appropriate forms and format.				
	H. Accurately classifies assigned patients using Patient Classification Index.				
	II. Planning				
	A. Develops individualized nursing care plan for primary patients incorporating:				
	1. data base				
	2. cultural and psychosocial components				
	3. short- and long-term goals				
	4. medical plan of care				
	5. standards of care				
	6. learning needs of patient/significant others'				
	B. Collaborates with physician to facilitate coordination of patient care.				

P & P	REQUIRED COMPETENCIES	READ P & P	DEMO COMP	N.A.	COMMENTS
		DATE & INITIAL EACH ENTRY			
	Level I—Staff Nurse				
	C. Plans with patient/significant others to develop mutual goals and means for attaining.				
	D. Reviews nursing care plan with appropriate resource person(s).				
	E. Communicates plan of care to other health team members.				
	F. Initiates patient care conferences in order to elicit feedback and share patient care information.				
	G. Documents nursing care plan using appropriate form and format.				

Note: Thirteen pages of additional required competencies for the Level I Staff Nurse have been omitted.

LEVEL II—PRIMARY NURSE

1. *Policy:*

    Staff nurses may apply for advancement to Primary Nurse after three (3) months of employment at The Moses H. Cone Memorial Hospital. A qualified applicant may be hired as a Primary Nurse and must demonstrate ability to function under Primary Nurse job description and required competencies within three (3) months of employment. Staff nurses who can demonstrate the ability to function at Primary Nurse level job description and required competencies may apply to the Head Nurse by completing a Career Progression Review file. The promotion review process by the Head Nurse will allow for unsolicited peer recommendations of each candidate by fellow staff nurses. In the absence of the Head Nurse, application may be made to the Clinical Director. Promotion to or hiring as a Primary Nurse is subject to position availability.

2. *Procedure:*

    A. The Candidate:
    1. reviews own current practice to determine if Level II Primary Nurse career progression criteria are being met consistently.
    2. initiates the Career Progression Review process by completing a Career Progression Review file with the following data:
        a. Application form
        b. Curriculum vitae
        c. Current Performance Review (within one year)
        d. Completed required competencies for Primary Nurse in appropriate clinical area.
        e. Peer Recommendation(s)
        f. Copy of current CPR Certification as Basic Rescuer
        g. Personal and professional goals for Primary Nurse position
    3. submits completed Career Progression Review file to Head Nurse. A composite of all Peer Recommendations are provided upon candidate's request.

    B. The Head Nurse:
    1. posts notice of available positions and deadline for submission of Career Progression Review file.
    2. has the option to require additional solicited Peer Recommendation(s) to be included in candidate Progression Review file.
    3. reviews file for each candidate. Incomplete or inappropriate files are returned to applicant for revision.

4. interviews each candidate to review job performance, credentials, and goals.
5. posts names of all candidates one (1) week prior to review to allow for Unsolicited Peer Recommendations.
6. requests consultation with Clinical Director as needed.
7. discusses promotion decisions with Clinical Director and obtains approval.
8. notifies all candidates of results of promotion decision.
9. counsels candidates individually as needed.
10. notifies Clinical Director and Administrator of Nursing of promotion decision.
11. announces all promotions within the unit/clinical service.

CLINICAL CAREER TRACK: LEVEL II—PRIMARY NURSE

Required Competencies

The Required Competencies for the Clinical Career Track identify the nursing knowledge and skills expected at each level. It is expected that the nurse at any level be able to demonstrate the required competencies for all preceding levels. *Prior to promotion the nurse must demonstrate the required competencies* for the position being sought.

Key: P & P—policy and procedure reference
Read P & P—has read policy and procedure
Demo Comp—has demonstrated competency
N.A.—not applicable or not available in particular clinical specialty

P & P	REQUIRED COMPETENCIES	READ P & P	DEMO COMP	N.A.	COMMENTS
	Level II—Primary Nurse	DATE & INITIAL EACH ENTRY			
	I. Assessment				
	A. Exhibits proficiency and skill in the performance of assessment competencies as listed for the staff nurse.				
	B. Validates nursing care plan for accuracy and completeness for assigned patients.				
	C. Identifies patient needs for referral to resource services.				
	D. Assesses complex problems as related to assigned patients.				
	E. Applies the interpretation of diagnostic/monitoring data in the care of patients with complex health care problems.				
	II. Planning				
	A. Exhibits proficiency and skill in the performance of planning competencies as listed for staff nurse.				
	B. Consults with appropriate resource person(s) regarding development of nursing care plan when indicated.				

P & P	REQUIRED COMPETENCIES	READ P & P	DEMO COMP	N.A.	COMMENTS
		DATE & INITIAL EACH ENTRY			
	Level II—Primary Nurse				
	C. Assists in the development of standardized care plans and unit standards as requested.				
	D. Conducts patient care conferences in order to elicit feedback and share patient care information.				
	III. Implementation				
	A. Exhibits proficiency and skill in the implementation competencies listed for the staff nurse.				
	B. Maintains definable primary patient caseload.				
	C. Provides comprehensive nursing care to primary/associate patients.				
	D. Demonstrates advanced communication skills. 1. Demonstrates empathy in interactions with others.				
	2. Conducts patient care conferences.				

E. Serves as a resource person for staff in patient care delivery.					
F. Serves as a unit preceptor for the orientation of new employees.					
G. Assists other staff in: 1. problem solving.					
2. development of clinical skills.					
3. identification of learning needs.					
H. Assists in the implementation of patient/family educational programs.					
I. Demonstrates ability to function as charge nurse through assignment, coordination, and management of patient care.					
J. Assists in the revision of patient care policies/procedures/standards of care.					
K. Identifies and communicates problems/questions for clinical research.					

P & P	REQUIRED COMPETENCIES	READ P & P	DEMO COMP	N.A.	COMMENTS
	Level II—Primary Nurse	*DATE & INITIAL EACH ENTRY*			
	IV. Evaluation				
	A. Exhibits proficiency and skill in the performance of evaluation competencies as listed for the staff nurse.				
	B. Initiates appropriate measures to correct environmental safety hazards.				
	C. Evaluates achievement of professional goals and objectives.				
	D. Provides feedback to other health care givers based on observed patient responses.				

Note: Fourteen pages of descriptive information and required competencies for Level III Clinician and Level IV Clinical Specialist have been omitted.

PERFORMANCE EVALUATION

EMPLOYEE (NAME): _____   POSITION TITLE: <u>**PRIMARY NURSE**</u>
DEPARTMENT: _____   TIME IN POSITION: _____
SUPERVISOR (NAME): _____   EMPLOYMENT DATE: _____
SUPERVISOR (TITLE): _____

DATE OF LAST PERFORMANCE REVIEW: _____

Abbreviated Major Work Activities (Review the major work activities on the position description and use the key words to describe each area.) List major work activities in descending order of importance. Insert comments if performance is above or below Competent.

*(P or S)**	*Performance Rating*	*Comments*
1. (P) Accepts accountability for assigned patients on a 24-hr. basis by providing care when on duty and leaving instructions for other caregivers.		_____
2. (P) Utilizes the nursing process in providing care.		_____
3. (P) Assures adequate and effective discharge planning and teaching.		_____
4. (P) Holds other health care providers accountable for following plan of care & modifying when appropriate.		_____

* Next to the major work activity ( ) indicate if you consider it to be "Primary" (P) or "Secondary" (S)

Primary (P)—Most important results areas. Position must accomplish primary work activities to be effective. These primary areas are "make-or-break" aspects of the job.

Secondary (S)—These accountabilities support accomplishment of primary work activities.

5. (P) Communicates effectively
       with patient, family, and
       other health care providers.
6. (S) Shares knowledge and skill
       with other nurses
       appropriately.
7. (S) Participates in unit and/or
       departmental committees as
       appropriate.
8. (S) Assists with clinical
       research as requested.

9. ( ) _____

New England Medical Center

Boston

452 Beds

The Professional Development Program
The Concept and How It Works
Organizational Chart*

Staff Nurse—Inpatient
  Job Description
  Performance Appraisal**

---

*Department of Nursing, New England Medical Center, Boston, Mass.;
Sandra P. Twyon, R.N., M.S.N., Chairman.
**Developed by Kathleen A. Bower, R.N., M.S.N., Associate Chairman
of Nursing, for use by the Department of Nursing, New England Medical
Center, Boston, Mass.

THE PROFESSIONAL DEVELOPMENT PROGRAM

With the current shortage of nurses and, most remarkably, experienced nurses, NEMC is always looking for new ways to recruit and retain both the new graduate and the veteran nurses. In the past, NEMC has used a preceptorship program, continuing education programs, generous tuition reimbursement programs, and options of traditional and flexible time to attract nurses. These inducements are consistent with NEMC's acknowledgment of both the personal and professional needs of nurses. To complement this concept, a Professional Development Program (PDP) has been instituted to retain the NEMC staff nurse through job enrichment.

The PDP is a way of acknowledging and rewarding the NEMC nurse for professional accomplishments beyond the staff nurse job description. Professional tracks provide structure for professional development and advancement for the nurse who wishes "to remain at the bedside" without compelling her to pursue the managerial ladder. There will be as many nurses on professional tracks as successfully meet the accomplishment criteria. The accomplishments expected will reflect both the high level of nursing professionalism of which NEMC nurses are capable and the ideals and goals of NEMC for the 1980s.

The focus of professional nursing at NEMC has centered not only on direct patient care but also on the needs of the consumer; that is, education, research, and health care in his own community. As the professional nurse gains sophistication, the degree to which she implements these components of her role may be directly related to her own work satisfaction.

If nurses are truly to collaborate with other health providers, they must acknowledge and accept similar professional commitments in terms of education, research, and community concerns. By providing a structure of professional tracks, NEMC can help staff nurses to this level of professional activity. For these accomplishments, the NEMC nurse would receive both recognition and monetary rewards. These rewards are independent of merit, education, experience, or seniority.

THE CONCEPT AND HOW IT WORKS

The Philosophy

The framework on which the Professional Development Program is based is consistent with both the goals for the 1980s and the philosophy of the NEMC department of nursing. To complete any track, the nurse must demonstrate continual excellence as a staff nurse. This is the "nuts and bolts'' of the nursing philosophy. The accomplishments delineated by PDP clearly parallel the goals of the department and NEMC.

The development of a teaching program for either patients or staff by the nurse contributes to the NEMC commitment of teaching. Through research done by the nurse, the nursing knowledge base and the quality of patient care may be expanded and enhanced. Development of research, both medical and nursing, is a hospitalwide objective. Similarly, the health needs of the surrounding community can be met through the track requiring a community health project.

The structure for these accomplishments is designed to foster the opportunity for professional growth through individual, independent work.

The Process

The process through which the staff nurse achieves a Professional Development Track status begins with the nurse's initiative in meeting the established professional track criteria. First, the nurse must apply in writing to the PDP Board. This may be done in January, March, May, July and September of 1982 and quarterly thereafter. Application involves submitting in writing according to established guidelines, the project proposal. Once the project has been approved, it is implemented and maintained. Specific guidelines are available in the staff education office.

The responsibilities of the PDB Board are these. First, the Board must respond in writing to each application for candidacy within eight weeks of date of receipt. Acceptance is based on eligibility criteria and soundness of the project proposal. If the proposal is rejected, the candidate may submit another proposal before the next PDP acceptance deadline. Finally, on completion of the project, the Board reviews the breadth and quality of the work. If satisfactory, the candidate is awarded the new Professional Development Track status.

The Eligibility-for-Candidacy Criteria

These criteria must be met each time an applicant wishes to be considered for candidacy for either the first or later tracks:

1. The applicant must be a staff nurse or senior staff nurse.
2. The staff nurse must be employed a minimum of 32 hours per week for one year prior to applying for each track in the PDP.
3. The nurse must score above satisfactory on the most recent *staff nurse performance appraisal*. This assures that there is consistency

between the high quality of clinical performance and the high standards of the PDP.
4. The nurse must not have had any disciplinary action. This assures that professional tracks do not acknowledge nurses with behavior or performance problems.
5. The applicant must have satisfactory attendance record.

The Professional Development Program Board

This Board is the monitoring system for the PDP. The Board is composed of seven members: The Chairman of Nursing, the Nursing Department Organization Developer, one nonnurse from the NEMC Administration, and four nurse leaders, one of whom is Chairman. These people are responsible for accepting and rejecting proposals, for consulting with applicants, and evaluating the supporting mechanisms of the PDP.

Rewards for Achievement

Rewards for achievement are symbols of appreciation and are effective mechanisms to sustain positive performance. The achievements qualifying the nurse for advancement along the professional tracks are outstanding accomplishments. These contributions are "extras" beyond those normally expected of the average employee. Hence, a bonus reward is deemed appropriate for these achievements. At this time, for Track A, and each subsequent track, the nurse will be awarded $1,000 on completion of each step.

The purpose of this bonus system is to acknowledge excellence, to sustain the individual productive efforts, to retain the nurse at NEMC, and to motivate the nurse to even greater achievements.

Professional Development Track A

Professional track A is designed to enlarge the nurse's perspective of the entire institution. Activities expected are:

1. committee membership; and
2. development and implementation of a teaching program.

Committee membership allows the nurse to actively participate in hospital activities beyond the assigned unit. It also encourages nursing participation in the many facets of a health care delivery system.
A teaching program addresses the ongoing learning needs of a specific population of people at New England Medical Center. This program must

have clearly defined objectives, a management plan of implementation, and a stated means for evaluation. The teaching program must be completely developed and in full operation for nine months in order to meet the requirements of professional development track A.

At this time, specific guidelines for Professional Development Track A may be picked up by interested nurses in the Staff Education Department.

Professional Development Tracks B, C, and D

Professional development tracks B, C, and D are interchangeable. A nurse must first provide evidence of continuation of the teaching program that qualified her for track A. The nurse may then choose any of the following three projects:

1. Research;
2. Community Program; or
3. Publication.

The nurse advances to track B upon successful completion of one of these projects. With successful completion of two, the criteria for track C is satisfied. Upon completion of all three, the nurse earns the distinction of track D.

Guidelines for these projects are in the process of being developed.

NEW ENGLAND MEDICAL CENTER HOSPITAL
DEPARTMENT OF NURSING

JOB DESCRIPTION

Job Title: Staff Nurse—Inpatient

Reports to: Assistant Nurse Leader

General Description: Provides skilled, creative nursing care to patients in an acute environment. Actively participates as a member of the nursing staff.

Is Primary Nurse for a caseload of patients and:
—assesses the initial and ongoing patient needs and problems.
—formulates a list of patient needs and problems.
—develops long- and short-term goals.
—designs interventions to achieve the stated goals based on pathophysiological and psychosocial rationale.

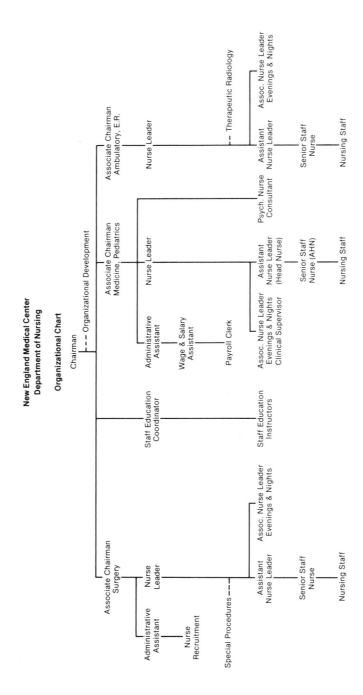

New England Medical Center
Department of Nursing

Organizational Chart

—implements the interventions.
—evaluates patient responses to care.
—modifies goals and interventions in response to changing patient needs.
—assists patients and their families in planning for discharge or transfer so that problems and needs are anticipated.
—provides patients and their families with the information they need to cope with their health situation.
—includes the patient's family in the plan of care.

Documents all aspects of patient care.

Assumes the charge role and:
—directs and supervises the care given by ancillary staff.
—manages the care of all patients on the unit for that shift.
—keeps the supervisory staff apprised of changing patient and unit conditions.
—anticipates the needs of the next shift.

Interacts with nursing staff as well as staff from other disciplines to:
—coordinate the patient's care with that planned by others.
—ensure continuity of care.
—interpret the nursing plan of care.

Provides direct patient care and:
—demonstrates excellent technical skills and judgment.
—administers medications, IVs, and treatments safely.
—maintains patient safety, comfort, and cleanliness.
—transcribes and implements physician orders accurately.

Effectively relates with:
—patients, their families, and visitors.
—nursing staff members.
—members of other disciplines and departments.
—introduces self as Primary Nurse to the nurse and explains the role.
—participates in and attends unit staff meetings.

Utilizes and provides peer support in providing care to primary patients.
—delegates specific aspects of patient care to colleagues during the absence of the Primary Nurse.
—presents patients during primary nursing conferences.
—uses the expertise of the unit nursing staff and the supervisory staff in dealing with patient care problems.

Participates in educational activities including:
—unit and institutional conferences, workshops, and forums.

—selected participation in the preceptor program.
—presentation of educational and primary nursing conferences.
—reading current nursing and related literature.
—maintenance of an on-unit record of educational activities.

Qualifications: Current Massachusetts license.
                Experience in the area of desired position preferred.
                Baccalaureate degree in nursing or diploma preferred.

KB/pt
2/6/80
Copyright, 1980 NEMCH

Return to Chairman's   3 Month _____
Office by _____

                                      6 Month _____
                NEW ENGLAND MEDICAL   Annual _____
                    CENTER HOSPITAL   Merit _____
            DEPARTMENT OF NURSING   Other _____
                                      Self _____

**PERFORMANCE APPRAISAL OF
INPATIENT STAFF NURSE**

NAME _____ DATE OF EMPLOYMENT _____
UNIT _____ DATE OF EVALUATION _____

There are two categories of evaluation criteria. One consists of single statements, each worth 3 points. No partial credit may be given. The other category consists of multiple statements of which one is to be selected. ($a = 3$, $b = 2$, $c = 1$, $d = 0$) Indicate the statement that best describes the usual performance of the employee.

A. GENERAL RESPONSIBILITIES AS A PRIMARY NURSE:

1. Thoroughly and accurately assesses the initial and ongoing patient needs and problems.   _____
2. Formulates a comprehensive set of patient needs and problems as indicated in the Nursing Index.   _____
3. Develops realistic and appropriate long- and short-term goals.   _____
4. Designs specific interventions to achieve the established goals and indicates them on the care plan.   _____
5. Implements the care plan.   _____

6. Patient treatment records reflect current needs and orders. _____

7. Evaluates and records patient responses to care. _____

8. Modifies goals and interventions in response to changing patient needs. _____

9. Assists patients and their families in planning for discharge or transfer so that problems and care needs are anticipated. _____

DOCUMENTATION OF PATIENT CARE:

10. Accurately depicts the patient's current status. _____
11. Indicates the patient's response to nursing care. _____
12. Demonstrates movement toward achievement of goals. _____
13. Summarizes the patient's status on transfer or discharge. _____
14. Is provided for other patients in the absence of their Primary Nurse. _____
15. Follows established guidelines. _____

TOTAL POSSIBLE POINTS: 45

B. PROFESSIONAL RELATIONSHIPS

*1. Approach to the patient is sensitive and courteous. _____

2. Introduces self as the primary nurse and explains responsibilities to the patient and family. _____

3. Is courteous and helpful to all unit personnel. _____

4. Communicates goals and plans for care to staff from other disciplines and other nursing staff members to enhance continuity and coordination. _____

5. The patient and family are included in care and its planning. _____

6. Utilizes and provides peer support in providing care to primary patients. _____

7. a) Evaluates own performance and seeks validation resulting in a positive change in behavior. _____

   b) Utilizes constructive criticism to affect an appropriate positive change in behavior. _____

   c) Accepts constructive criticism and there is a temporary positive change in behavior that must be periodically reinforced. _____

* Refer to last page.

*d) Denies a need for constructive criticism and/or demonstrates no positive change in behavior. _____

8. a) Uses insight into effect of own behavior on others to successfully control reactions that would be detrimental to patient care or interdepartmental relationships and to foster positive relationships. _____

   b) Can describe how behavior affects others but requires help in handling problem situations. _____

   c) Requires assistance to develop insight into the effect of own behavior on patient, staff, or interdepartmental relationships. _____

   *d) Consistently demonstrates inappropriate behavior despite counselling. _____

9. a) Impresses patients with sincerity and concern for their care. Maintains a professional yet personable relationship with patients that enhances the identification and fulfillment of patient needs. Exceeds expected efforts to enhance meaningful communication and patient's comfort. _____

   b) Is courteous with patients and maintains a professional relationship in which patient needs can be identified and met. Does not go beyond overt needs. _____

   c) Maintains a casual relationship with patients that may not always provide for identification and resolution of patient problems. _____

   *d) Cannot maintain a professional relationship with the patient and/or patients complain that the nurse is rude and abrupt with them or unconcerned about meeting their needs. _____

10. a) Seeks out concerns or fears that the patient needs or wants to discuss and is able to establish a relationship that enhances communication. _____

   b) Readily discusses the patient's overt fears or concerns in a "situation-limited" relationship, but fails to explore underlying emotional needs. _____

   c) Is oblivious to the patient's need to talk about fears or concerns, but accepts guidance in developing an approach to the resolution of these fears and concerns once identified. _____

---

* Refer to last page.

*d) Rejects or ignores the patient who has fears or concerns needing verbalization. _____

_____
TOTAL POSSIBLE POINTS: 30
_____

C. MANAGEMENT OF PATIENT CARE
Makes assignments that:
1. Provide for all work to be done. _____
2. Consider each worker's preparation, ability, or need for experience. _____
3. Consider the needs and problems of each patient. _____

Holds personnel accountable for assigned work by:
4. Clearly outlining expectations of staff at the beginning of the shift. _____
5. Observing the patients and the progress of their care periodically during the shift. _____
6. Obtaining a report from each staff member before the end of the shift. _____

Provides for a smooth intershift transition by:
7. Beginning and ending report on time. _____
8. Giving a patient report to the next shift following the specified guidelines. _____
9. Anticipating and providing for the patient care activities of the next shift. _____
10. Leaving the patient's environment clean and in order. _____
11. When in a position of authority communicates with personnel in a manner that is considerate but maintains control of assignments, thus holding personnel accountable for patient care. _____
*12. Assumes the charge role and manages the unit smoothly for that shift. _____
13. Keeps supervisory staff appraised of changing patient or unit conditions. _____
14. Adjusts assignments and priorities in response to a changing work load, considering the needs of all patients. Communicates these changes to necessary staff members so all will be aware of the new expectations. _____

_____

* Refer to last page.

15. a) Priorities and decisions concerning patient care are safe and ensure that multilevel needs for a group of patients as well as the individual patient will be met. _____

   b) Priorities and decisions about patient care are safe and ensure that safety and basic care needs for a group of patients as well as the individual patient will be met. Requires guidance to meet higher level needs. _____

   c) Priorities established for the individual patient are safe and address basic needs. Requires guidance to meet the needs of a group of patients. _____

   *d) Priorities established in decisions about patient care are unsafe and require constant supervision and guidance. _____

16. a) Organizational skills enable the nurse to complete assigned work, thereby providing extra time to spend with patients and to assist fellow staff members. _____

   b) Organizational skills enable the nurse to complete assigned work by the end of the shift. _____

   c) Organizational skills enable the nurse to complete assigned workload but requires guidance and supervision to ensure this is done. _____

   *d) Organization of work does not allow for completion of assigned workload and must be assisted by others to complete the assignment. _____

17. a) Assumes responsibility for the effective functioning of the total unit at all times. _____

   b) Assumes responsibility for the effective functioning of the total unit when in charge. _____

   c) Fulfills responsibility for effective functioning of assigned areas of the unit. _____

   d) Others must assume responsibility for the effective functioning of the total unit, including assigned areas. _____

TOTAL POSSIBLE POINTS: 51

---

* Refer to last page.

D. JUDGMENT

  1. a) Is observant of subtle as well as overt changes in the patient's condition that indicate an emerging problem. Relates these changes to a pathophysiological/psychological base and, using all available, relevant information, takes appropriate preventative, restorative, or emergency actions.

      b) Is observant of overt changes in patient's condition that indicate a problem has emerged and reports these changes to an appropriate person. Can anticipate equipment and medication that will be needed to control the situation. Needs assistance to observe, then act upon, subtle changes. _____

      c) Is observant of overt changes in patient's condition that indicate a problem has emerged. Reports these changes to the appropriate person. Awaits direction to take action that will control the situation. _____

   *d) Is unobservant of overt changes in patient's condition. _____

  2. a) Independently researches unfamiliar procedures, diseases, medications, and use of equipment. Uses this in making decisions that are confirmed as necessary. _____

      b) Independently researches unfamiliar procedures, diseases, medications, and use of equipment. Often needs assistance in making decisions. _____

      c) Asks for assistance when using unfamiliar equipment and medications. Does not usually do independent research. _____

   *d) Fails to research unfamiliar procedures, equipment, diseases, medications and does not seek assistance. This lends itself to situations where unsafe decisions may result. _____

  3. a) Independently makes and acts on judgments and decisions that promote the patient's well-being. Collaborates as necessary. _____

---

* Refer to last page.

b) Makes judgments and decisions that promote the patient's well-being but must often confirm them before they are enacted.   _____

c) Makes decisions and judgments that do not endanger the patient's health in any way but may not always consider all needs of the patient.   _____

*d) Decisions and judgments are unsound and may endanger the patient's health.   _____

4. Decisions about patient or family requests are made in light of sound practice and communicated promptly yet considerately. Alternatives are explored.   _____

TOTAL POSSIBLE POINTS: 12

E. TECHNICAL SKILLS

*1. Patients and their environment are clean, comfortable, and safe.   _____

2. Obtains and records patient data accurately and promptly.   _____

3. Positions and mobilizes in an anatomically correct and comfortable manner.   _____

4. Utilizes principles of asepsis in all patient contact.   _____

*5. Safely uses equipment common to the assigned clinical area.   _____

6. Utilizes appropriate measures for patient safety.   _____

*7. Physician's orders are transcribed accurately.   _____

8. Physician's orders are carried out promptly.   _____

Performs treatments and patient care activities:

9. On time.   _____

*10. Safely, following prescribed techniques.   _____

Medication Administration

*11. Administers medications and IVs safely by following the established procedures.   _____

12. Computes doses correctly.   _____

13. Medications are given within specified time limits.   _____

14. Does narcotic count with nurse from previous and oncoming shifts when responsible for medications.   _____

---

* Refer to last page.

15. Uses knowledge about usual doses, actions, and toxicology when making decisions regarding medication administration.   _____

TOTAL POSSIBLE POINTS: 45

F. TEACHING SKILLS

Patient Teaching

1. Assesses the learning needs of each Primary Patient and family considering the disease process, treatment plan, discharge needs, or other problems.   _____
2. Plans specific measures to meet the assessed learning needs.   _____
3. Utilizes appropriate audiovisual resources such as pictures or pamphlets.   _____
4. Presents appropriate information clearly and in a manner appropriate to the level of the patient or family.   _____
5. Evaluates the effectiveness of teaching activities.   _____
6. Updates and follows through on teaching that has been initiated.   _____
7. Documents the plan for teaching and the patient's response.   _____
8. Provides and documents necessary patient teaching in the absence of the primary nurse.   _____

Other Teaching Situations

9. Attends staff development conferences on a regular basis.   _____
10. Maintains an accurate on-unit record of own educational activities.   _____

Conducts Conferences for Other Staff Members That:

11. Present accurate and up-to-date information.   _____
12. Present the information in a clear and organized manner.   _____
13. Presents Primary Patients during Primary Nursing Conferences or Supervision.   _____

14. Assists in the orientation process by providing information or instruction and by making new staff feel welcome on the unit.   _____

TOTAL POSSIBLE POINTS: 42

G. GENERAL WORK HABITS

*1. Begins work on time.   _____
2. Stays until shift is ended.   _____
*3. Has not been conferenced for disciplinary problem within the last six months.   _____
4. Does not routinely call in ill or absent before or after a day off.   _____
5. Has had no unapproved absent days within the last six months.   _____
6. Is neat and well groomed.   _____
7. Wears name pin and school pin at all times while on duty.   _____
8. Answers call lights as they appear and/or responds to patient's requests promptly.   _____
9. Willingly provides assistance to other nursing units when requested to do so by the supervisor or charge nurse.   _____
10. Equally shares the responsibility for overtime and necessary schedule changes with other nurses on the unit.   _____

TOTAL POSSIBLE POINTS: 30

A. NARRATIVE SUMMARY OF PERFORMANCE

1. Areas Requiring Improvement

* Refer to last page.

2. Areas of Strength

B. SPECIFIC PLANS AND GOALS FOR THE NEXT EVALUATION PERIOD.

C. CURRENT PERFORMANCE STATUS.

    1.—Did the employee receive a "0" on any asterisked (*) statements?
        Yes _____ No _____
    —If no, proceed to the next step.
    —If yes, please turn to section entitled probationary/termination status. Do not complete the rating section (2B); only calculate total points earned.

    2. A. Enter the total points earned for each category. Calculate total.

	A	B	C	D	E	F	G	Total
POSSIBLE POINTS	45	30	51	12	45	42	30	255
POINTS EARNED								

B. Check appropriate scale. Indicate rating according to total points
   earned.

Rating	☐ 3 & 6 Month	☐ 12 To 60 Month	☐ 2 Months & Above	
Above Average	( ) 229-255	( ) 241-255	5%	241-255 ( )
Satisfactory	( ) 178-228	( ) 190-240	3%	206-240 ( )
*Probation	( ) 139-177	( ) 152-189	0%	190-205 ( )
*Termination	( ) 0-138	( ) 0-151	Probation	152-189 ( )
			Termination	0-151 ( )

EVALUATOR (Signature & Title) _____ DATE _____

ASSISTANT NURSE LEADER _____ DATE _____

NURSE LEADER _____ DATE _____

ASSOCIATE NURSE LEADER _____ DATE _____
(must sign permanent shift employee's evaluation)

COMMENTS BY EMPLOYEE: (Use additional page as necessary)

*EMPLOYEE'S SIGNATURE _____ DATE _____
* Indicates only that employee has read report; does not imply agreement.

PROBATIONARY/TERMINATION STATUS

1. Describe in specific terms the problems resulting in the status of pro-
   bation or termination.

2. Outline the specific behaviors that must be demonstrated in order for
   removal of the *Probationary Status*.

3. Indicate the length of the *Probationary Status* _____
Date

   If termination, indicate the last day of work _____

4. Course of action if behaviors outlined in step 2 are not successfully demonstrated during the Probationary Period.

5. Written, weekly conference reports are required throughout the probationary status.

KAB/pt
2/4/80
Copyright, 1980 NEMCH

Presbyterian Hospital of Pacific Medical Center

San Francisco

433 Beds

Job Description: Food Service Director

Reprinted by permission of Kenneth Petron, Director, Personnel Services.

PACIFIC MEDICAL CENTER JOB DESCRIPTION

Job Title __Food Service Director__   Account # __8320__ Date _____
Job Code __078__ Class Code ____   Department ____Food Service____
Exempt __X__ Non Exempt ____   Personnel Approval _____

PRIMARY PURPOSE OF JOB: The overall purpose or key objective of this position is to contribute to the efficient and cost-effective operation of the total hospital patient care system by providing or causing to be provided essential and cost-effective food service that enhances patient care and patient comfort. The Food Director shall ensure that the principles of the science of nutrition are applied to the preparation of palatable and appropriate food.

LEVEL OF AUTHORITY:
   (A) Full Authority   (B) Act and Report   (C) Approval, then act

Major Responsibilities	*Performance Standards*	*Level of Authority*
To Director of Support Services:		
1. Assess plan, assure implementation, and evaluate the activities of the department. (JCAH-I)	1. Quality service to patients and staff is maintained.	B
2. Assess needs, establish long-range and short-range goals for the department. (JCAH-I)	2. Goals are in writing. Results are evaluated.	B
3. Plan and organize the budget needs of the department. (JCAH-I)	3. Budget approval is obtained.	B&C
4. Establish and maintain orientation and training programs for food service employees. (JCAH-II, Title 22-70275 C)	4. Subjects required are understood by employees.	B
5. Develop, revise, update, and assure implementation of policies and procedures both for intra and interdepartmental activities. (JCAH-III)	5. Policies and procedures are understood by all concerned.	B

6. Participate in department head committee and interdepartmental meetings as a member. (JCAH-I)

6. Input is accepted and understood.   B

7. Provide liaison between Administration and the department. (JCAH-I)

7. Keep your boss well informed.   B&C

8. Recruit, select, and appoint personnel to the food service department. Promote, disqualify, terminate, discipline, and counsel food service employees. (JCAH-I, Title 22-70275)

8. Best trainable personnel are hired. Files are maintained on disciplinary problems.   A

9. Participate in professional organizations as the hospital's representative liaison. (JCAH-II)

9. Actively support the hospital's position at these meetings.   A&B

10. Study, evaluate, and introduce new methods, equipment, and materials, participate in planning physical facility changes of the food service department. (JCAH-I)

10. Make recommendations to Administration. Employees understand and are a part of the change.   B&C

To Patients and Patrons:
1. Prepare all menus in conjunction with Senior Dietitian, taking into consideration availability of supplies, equipment and personnel. (JCAH-III-45)

1. Menus prepared in accordance with 4 basic food groups are productively possible, economically feasible, and meet budget restrictions.   B

2. Estimate quantities and order all perishable supplies, ensure par controls are followed for ordering nonperishable supplies. (JCAH-III-40, Title 22-70277)

2. Order only what is needed on menu. Use census and recipes for determining amounts of perishables.   A

LEVEL OF AUTHORITY:

(A) Full Authority   (B) Act and Report   (C) Approval, then act

Major Responsibilities	*Performance Standards*	*Level of Authority*
3. Establish portion controls and ensure that portion cost effectiveness is maintained. Inspect and schedule the use of all left-overs to prevent waste, and comply with sanitation requirements. (JCAH-IV, Title 22-70273)	3. Procedures are in writing and posted. Waste is kept to a minimum.	A

To Employees

Major Responsibilities	*Performance Standards*	*Level of Authority*
1. Frequently evaluate work performance and work assignments of food service personnel. (JCAH-I, Title 22-70279)	1. Evaluate and update job descriptions as necessary. Evaluate and make recommendations for adequate staffing, reducing labor costs whenever possible.	B
2. Plan personal hygiene programs for food service employees. (JCAH-II, Title 22-70273, 22-70275)	2. Employees keep a neat and clean appearance at all times.	A
3. Ensure constant effective supervision is maintained over all phases of sanitation procedures. (Title 22-70203-1)	3. Procedures are written and posted. Environmental diseases are controlled.	
4. Establish and evaluate effectiveness of departmental safety program. (JCAH-IV, Title 22-70277)	4. Investigate all industrial accidents. Take corrective action if possible. Involve employees in group discussion.	B
5. Identify problems, resolve problems using professional knowledge, questioning and listening techniques. (JCAH-I-15)	5. Problems are identified and resolved to everyone's satisfaction as much as possible.	ABC

6. Solicit cooperation, promote and maintain harmonious relationships among food service personnel and other departments of hospital. Make effective decisions to resolve misunderstandings and inconsistencies. (JCAH-I)

6. Good working relationship with others in department are maintained.   A & B

St. John's Hospital

Red Wing, Minn.

88 Beds

Nursing Supervisor Performance Evaluation Form

Reprinted by permission of Ruth A. Erickson, Director of Nursing.

NURSING SUPERVISOR PERFORMANCE EVALUATION

Name _____ Title _____ Date _____ Evaluator _____

Performance Accountability	Standard	Performance Evaluation
To:		
A. *Director of Nursing*		
1. Functions within and supports the general policies, beliefs, and philosophy of St. John's Hospital & the Dept. of Nsg.	1. Such is demonstrated through verbalization & behavior.	
2. Communicates information regarding policies & procedures to staff appropriately.	2. Evidence of communication exists (i.e., staff following revised policy).	
3. Participates in staffing policy development and implementation.	3. Communicates policies to staff & enforces policies as appropriate. Corrective action taken when necessary.	
4. Assists with daily adjustments in staffing based on changing needs.	4. Adjustments are made with good judgment and daily assignment of personnel is appropriate. NA is informed promptly of all changes.	
5. Keeps Director or Assistant informed regarding personnel problems or concerns regarding unit activity.	5. Nursing Administration does not experience many "surprises."	

6. Seeks assistance from Director or Assistant in resolving management problems.

7. Participates with Nursing Administration in data collection and research programs within the nursing department.

8. Maintains good interpersonal relationships with other departments.

9. Works cooperatively with Nursing Administration in budget planning, control, and evaluation.

B. *To Nursing Units*

1. Acts as a consultant and management role model for Head Nurse & Unit Supervisors.

2. Provides general supervision, & observation/assessment of daily unit operation. Assists unit manager with problem solving as necessary.

6. Evidence exists that this type of communication takes place.

7. Evidence of cooperation, such as reports, accurate statistics, and data requested are available. Serves on committees as appointed.

8. Evidence of cooperation exists. Problems are resolved or referred to Nursing Administration as appropriate.

9. Demonstrates concern for cost effective utilization of staff and materials. Communicates this to staff supervised.

1. Demonstrates skill in communicating management functions & techniques.

2. Rounds are made regularly. Problems are identified & solutions developed cooperatively. Demonstrates skill in use of problem-solving technique.

Performance Accountability	Standard	Performance Evaluation
3. Evaluates work performance & prepares annual performance evaluation report for staff directly supervised.	3. Guidance and constructive discipline are used appropriately. Evaluations are completed when due.	
4. Arranges for supplies & equipment as needed when other departments are not staffed.	4. Obtains pharmacy items, CSR, linen, or other supplies as needed and keeps accurate records.	
C. *To Patient and Family*		
1. Provides or arranges for the immediate needs of the patient on admission.	1. Room assignments are generally appropriate. Physicians' admitting orders are completed & communicated.	
2. Is skilled in nursing assessment and can provide appropriate emergency care.	2. Systematic assessment is documented. Ability to perform under pressure is observable.	
3. Is aware of all resources available within the hospital and utilizes these appropriately.	3. Code Blue is used when indicated. Auxiliary services are utilized.	
4. Delegates responsibility for ER care & procedures to others according to patient needs and staff competency.	4. Evidence exists that delegation is used appropriately & accountability is maintained. Pt. needs are met.	

D. *To Medical Staff*

1. Acts as liaison between physician and patient care team.

   1. Medical care plan is communicated to nursing unit and other departments.

2. Receive, transcribe, communicate, and assist with interpretation and implementation of medical care plan.

   2. Physicians' orders are accurately carried out. Orders are questioned when not clear.

3. Acts as resource to physicians regarding hospital policies & procedures.

   3. Policies & procedures are known and followed. Problems are identified and referred appropriately.

4. Schedules procedures. Maintains accurate records of ER activities.

   4. Methods are developed and implemented to allow efficient daily operation of the department. Records are complete. Statistics are accurate.

5. Assists with procedures through appropriate use of staff, equipment, and supplies.

   5. Effective & efficient use of resources is evident.

E. *To Self*

1. Is knowledgeable of health care trends and changes in nursing.

   1. Participates in appropriate professional organizations.

2. Assumes personal responsibility for continuing educa-

   2. Level of skill required is maintained.

Performance Accountability	Standard	Performance Evaluation
tion and professional development.		
3. As a member of the nursing department management team, recognizes need for increased skill in management as well as nursing.	3. Demonstrates competence in planning, organizing, directing, and evaluating nursing care and staff performance.	

EVALUATION CONFERENCE

Employee Comments:

Personal or Professional Goals:

Employee Signature _____ Evaluator Signature _____ Date _____

St. Mary's Hospital

Milwaukee

300 Beds

Career Ladder Application Process
R.N. Career Ladder Outline and Time Frame
Clinical Nurse Performance Appraisal

Reprinted by permission of Marjorie P. Davis, Assistant Administrator.

St. Mary's Hospital

NURSING DEPARTMENT

CAREER LADDER APPLICATION PROCESS

The Career Ladder Application Process is designed to allow R.N.s to demonstrate nursing competency and readiness for promotion. To facilitate the Application Process you are requested to compile a folder with inclusions that demonstrate your nursing competency.

All forms may be obtained in Nursing Service.

As you submit completed documents they will be placed in your folder for review by the Nurse Practice Committee.

Inclusions for Career Ladder Application Folder:

I. Complete the Letter of Intent to Seek Promotion with your Supervisor and return to Nursing Service.

II. On a separate sheet of paper submit a personal statement describing your qualifications. (Personal and Professional) that indicate readiness for promotion.

This can include areas of Clinical Expertise (technical, psychosocial, and teaching skills):

A. Professional organization memberships.
B. Special achievements/certifications.
C. *List of CEUs obtained in past year.
D. *Date of last CPR certification.
E. Professional contributions to the community.
F. Participation in nursing/hospital committee work.
G. Involvement in planning and/or presentation of staff development programs; e.g., Grand Rounds, Unit-Based classes.
H. Patient/staff education materials developed or shared with Unit or Quad staff.
I. Examples of patient/staff education materials developed or shared with Quad/Unit staff.
J. *Staff development classes or workshops attended within the past year.
K. List of Unit Meetings attended within the past year.
L. List of Quad Meetings attended within the past year.

AND

---

* Call and request the Nursing Education Secretary (Ext. 7096) to place a copy of your Nursing Education Record in your folder.

For Nurse III Applications

M. Statement of involvement in orientation of new staff.
N. Examples of formal/informal counseling of staff.
O. Management activities on quad (coordination of hours, supervision of L.P.N., N.A., communication of problems to Unit Supervisor).
P. Quality Assurance activities on Quad.

III. Documentation of Clinical Nursing Practice.

A. Copies of two Care Plans of primary patients with complex needs cared for within the past three months.
B. Copy of a comprehensive teaching plan for a patient cared for within the past three months (may be part of Care Plan from Part A above).
C. Copy of critique by peer(s) from Patient Care Conference held within the past twelve months.
D. Clinical Nurse III on Quad or Unit.

IV. Include a statement of your philosophy of Primary Nursing.

V. Submit a Letter of Recommendation. (Form Letters are kept in Nurs. Service)

A. Unit Supervisor
B. PM/N Supervisor
C. Clinical Specialist
D. Clinical Nurse III on Quad or Unit

VI. Attendance Calendar Data for previous 18 months will be supplied by the Staffing Office.

1/13/82 lmt

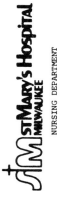

ST MARY'S HOSPITAL
MILWAUKEE

NURSING DEPARTMENT

RN CAREER LADDER OUTLINE AND TIMEFRAME

Required RN Experience	CLINICAL	Required RN Experience	EDUCATIONAL + MANAGEMENT	Required RN Experience	ADMINISTRATIVE
0-1 year	CLINICAL NURSE I				
18 months	CLINICAL NURSE II				
2 years	CLINICAL NURSE III (Clinician)	3 years →	· CENTRAL INSTRUCTOR (BSN) · Q. A. COORDINATOR (BSN) · UNIT SEC. SUPERVISOR (BSN) · ASSISTANT SUPERVISOR (BSN) (Unit, PM/N)		
5 years	CLINICAL SPECIALIST (MSN)	5 years	NURSING EDUC. COORDINATOR (MSN)	5 years	PM/N SUPERVISOR (BSN)
				6 years	UNIT SUPERVISOR (BSN)
				7 years	ASSISTANT DIRECTOR (MSN) · Clin. Practice/ED · Nurs. Resources/QA
				10 years	ASST. ADMINISTRATOR/NSG (MSN)

9/81

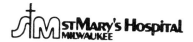

CLINICAL NURSE PERFORMANCE APPRAISAL

Name	Department/Cost Center
Title (Encircle One)	Appraisal Period/Due Date:
Clinical Nurse I, II, III	6 mos. _____ Annual _____ Term _____ Other _____

PURPOSE: This appraisal is an important part of the employee's relationship with
St. Mary's Hospital - for this reason it should be a mutually participative review
between the employee and the rater. The appraisal serves to 1) encourage continued
successful performance and strengthen weaknesses, 2) evaluate the nurse's contribution
to patient care, and 3) identify and prepare individuals for increased responsibilities.

DIRECTIONS: Each competency is judged by scoring several performance criteria. The
scores within a competency are averaged. Minimal acceptance performance is an average
score of 2.0 for each competency. Clinical Nurse I's are scored in the first level;
Clinical Nurse II's are scored in the first two levels; Clinical Nurse III's are scored
in all three levels. Written communication comment space is provided following each of
the six competencies. Attendance as an additional measure and a profile of the evaluation
are recorded on the final pages.

RATING:

4. Outstanding: Far exceeds a satisfactory level of performance.
3. Satisfactory: Consistently meets performance expectations.
2. Marginal: At, or slightly above the minimum level of performance.
1. Unsatisfactory: Not meeting the minimal expected level of performance.
   N.A.: Not applicable (write in - NO SCORE/omit in calculation).

A [   ]   NURSING PROCESS: This is an appraisal of how effectively the nurse utilizes
                the elements of the Nursing Process (assessment, diagnosis, planning,
                implementation and evaluation).

Level   Rating   Performance Criteria

  I   _____ 1. Documentation included in the nursing admission assessment reflects
                     knowledge of patient's physiological status through physical assessment.
         _____ 2. Documentation included in the foregoing reflects knowledge of the
                     patient's psychosocial status.
         _____ 3. Develops problem list from initial assessment and data obtained from
                     patient/family.
         _____ 4. Utilizes appropriate nursing diagnosis to identify care problems and
                     develop strategies for outcomes.
         _____ 5. Determines the need for ongoing assessments and records schedule on the
                     nursing care plan.
         _____ 6. Documents patient responses to care regimes (medical and nursing).
                     Revises as indicated.
         _____ 7. Consults resources when confronted with a new or unfamiliar task or
                     situation and follow through effectively.
         _____ 8. Identifies the following common behavioral responses to illness or role
                     change: anger, denial, depression, grief, anxiety, non-compliance.

(÷ by 8)

A. NURSING PROCESS (continued)

Level	Rating		Performance Criteria
II	____	9.	Identifies signs and symptoms which indicate potential physiologic problems; correlates these with abnormalities found in the data base; further, takes action which reflects knowledge and good judgment (implies consultation with Medical Staff and Nursing Administration).
	____	10.	Plans effective strategies and time frames for achieving desired patient outcomes.
	____	11.	Assists Clinical Nurse I's and LPN's in foregoing.
	____	12.	Coordinates the medical and the nursing plans of care.
	____	13.	Assists Clinical Nurse I's in identifying strategies to deal with behavioral responses to illness.

(÷ by 13)

Level	Rating		Performance Criteria
III	____	14.	Demonstrates skill in handling complex patient care situations.
	____	15.	Evaluates nursing care at the quad level on a planned basis with other Clinical Nurse III's.

(÷ by 15)

Comments (Nursing Process)

B [____] **HUMAN RELATIONS:** This is a measure of human relations skills and personal characteristics associated with job performance. It includes attitude plus oral and written communication skills with patients, peers, physicians, other health team members and supervisor.

Level	Rating		Performance Criteria
I		1.	Documentation follows the POMR format guidelines (Nursing Procedure Manual).
	____	A.	Documents appropriately on chart forms.
	____	B.	Demonstrates an understanding of the legal implications of charting.
	____	C.	Charts within an acceptable time frame.
	____	2.	Demonstrates effective interviewing skills with patients and/or family and friends (gaining information necessary to plan, implement, and evaluate nursing care).
	____	3.	Applies basic verbal and non-verbal communication skills to identify and reduce patient anxiety (and/or family/friends).
	____	4.	Interacts effectively with the Medical Staff, other members of the health team, and other departmental personnel.
	____	5.	Verbalizes patient care expected outcomes and care strategies to co-workers in change of shift report and throughout the shift.
		6.	Communicates "Primary Nursing" by:
	____	A.	Explaining care model to patient/family (Primary Nurse Card).
	____	B.	Listing self as P.N. on Care Plan, Primary Board, Hollister.
	____	7.	Maintains confidentiality of information.

(÷ by 10)

B. HUMAN RELATIONS (continued)

Level Rating   Performance Criteria

II   ____   8. Promotes quad/unit cohesiveness through positive peer support and care
                     group direction (RN I's, LPN's, NA's).
          ____   9. Communicates information about staff's needs to appropriate person.

(÷ by 12)

III   ____ 10. Assists other staff members with difficult or complex communication
                     with Medical Staff, patients, and families.
          ____ 11. Holds quad meetings in conjunction with other Clinical Nurse III's
                     (as delegated by supervisor).
          ____ 12. Advocates and assists quad staff in the presentation of patient care
                     conferences on an ongoing basis.
          ____ 13. Monitors the quad bulletin boards and all posted material on a regular
                     basis (as delegated by supervisor).
          ____ 14. Assists in resolution of staff conflict.
          ____ 15. Submits periodic reports to the supervisor as scheduled on a timely basis.
          ____ 16. Refers management problems to supervisor promptly.

(÷ by 19)

Comments (Human Relations)

C   _____   QUALITY ASSURANCE: This is a measure of the individual's professional
               commitment to the process of evaluation of patient care. It includes safety
               measures and adherence to standards and policies/procedures.

Level Rating   Performance Criteria

I   ____   1. Adheres to established nursing policies, procedures, and standards of care.
          ____   2. Utilizes nursing quality assurance resource manual to plan care based upon
                     nursing standards.
          ____   3. Assists in identifying and resolving actual or potential patient care
                     problems.
          ____   4. Demonstrates the ability to assess basic safety needs of patients in
                     consultation with appropriate resources.

(÷ by 4)

II   ____   5. Demonstrates skill in planning care for patients with complex safety needs.
          ____   6. Assists Nurse I's, LPN's, NA's in translating standards of care into an
                     effective plan of care for the patient.
                 7. Actively participates in the Nursing QA Program.
          ____   A. Completes concurrent audits as assigned.
          ____   B. Participates on Nursing QA and/or Safety Committees as requested.
          ____   8. Participates in the peer review process.
          ____   9. Identifies effective methods for resolving patient care problems.

(÷ by 10)

C. QUALITY ASSURANCE: (continued)

Level	Rating	Performance Criteria
III	10.	Evaluates the effectiveness of care on a periodic basis by:
	A.	Reviewing Nursing Care Plans with Level I, II RN's.
	B.	Monitoring the care environment.
	C.	Auditing patient data relative to area (incidents, QA reports, patient evaluation feedback).
	11.	Values and encourages the contribution of quad/unit personnel which promotes group problem solving.
	12.	Promotes commitment to nursing quality assurance through active participation in clinician section meetings, workshops, unit meetings, etc.
	13.	Participates in the development of written standards, unit and/or quad goals plus demonstrates effective action toward implementation.

(÷ by 16)

Comments (Q.A.)

D

LEADERSHIP AND DECISION MAKING: These criteria measure the professional nurse's leadership role inherent in the Primary Nurse Model of care delivery; decision making reflects use of the nursing process.

Level	Rating	Performance Criteria
I	1.	Fulfills Primary or Associate Nurse role and maintains a primary case load (exception - permanent night shift).
	2.	Delegates patient care activities to appropriate care personnel consistent with State Licensure Law and Nursing policy.
	3.	Interfaces effectively with the nursing students obtaining clinical experience in the area.
	4.	Recognizes and takes immediate action in crisis situations.
	5.	Decisions reveal values consistent with Nursing and Hospital philosophy.

(÷ by 5)

Level	Rating	Performance Criteria
II	6.	Accepts accountability in the total assessment of nursing care of primary patients from admission to discharge.
	7.	Contributes to the cohesiveness of the quad/unit by assisting in goal setting and evaluation of care delivered.
	8.	Assists in the compilation of Monthly Hours Schedules/evaluates for employee needs/fairness and patient coverage guidelines.
	9.	Recognizes limitations of others and takes corrective action (as delegated by supervisor).
	10.	Evaluates effectiveness and implications of own decisions.

(÷ by 10)

D.   LEADERSHIP AND DECISION MAKING: (continued)

Level	Rating		Performance Criteria
III		11.	Functions as a Role Model in all aspects of Professional Practice within area of specialty.
		12.	Initiates and supports improvements for the quad/unit in procedure, policy and practice.
		13.	Provides feedback to quad personnel and to supervisor regarding nursing practice.
		14.	Selects leadership style appropriate to a given situation/event.
		15.	Interacts appropriately and effectively with supervisory personnel.
		16.	Delegates tasks effectively.

(÷ by 16)

Comments (Leadership/Decision Making)

E   [ ]   TEACHING/DISCHARGE PLANNING: This section measures the nurse's skill in assessing health needs of patients and in developing strategies for effective discharge of the patient. (In both areas, collaboration with the physician and other health team members is necessary).

Level	Rating		Performance Criteria
I		1.	Establishes written teaching/learning goals and objectives in collaboration with patient and family.
		2.	Assists patient and family to adapt to hospital environment.
		3.	Demonstrates basic knowledge of teaching/learning principles and is able to evaluate effectiveness of effort.
		4.	Initiates and carries out an effective discharge plan for primary patients.

(÷ by 4)

II		5.	Provides guidance to Clinical Nurse I's and LPN's in implementing an effective teaching/discharge plan.
		6.	Participates in the development of patient education materials in designated area.
		7.	Uses all available hospital resources to accomplish teaching/discharge goals.
		8.	Adapts teaching skills and plan to individual situations.

(÷ by 8)

III		9.	Coordinates and updates patient education materials in area.
		10.	Plans for quad/unit programs in collaboration with supervisor/assistant and other Clinicians toward increasing teaching skill of Staff Nurse I and II's.
		11.	Facilitates the health education of patients/families on an ongoing basis.

(÷ by 11)

Comments (Teaching/Discharge Planning)

F [   ]

PROFESSIONAL GROWTH: This area measures the nurse's own initiative and commitment to growth through active participation and involvement in ongoing nursing education programs.

Level	Rating		Performance Criteria
I	____	1.	Participates in formal self-evaluation by identifying areas of strengths and weaknesses and sets goals toward improvement.
	____	2.	Updates practice in accordance with changes in hospital/nursing policies and procedures.
	____	3.	Achieves CPR recertification annually.
	____	4.	Attends mandatory hospital/nursing sponsored inservice programs.
	____	5.	Accrues 1.2 CEU's annually. (OR EQUIVALENT).
	____	6.	Participates in unit business and staff development meetings - as outlined by supervisor.
	____	7.	Presents patient care conferences utilizing hospital resources (and takes responsibility for documentation of same).

(÷ by 7)

Level	Rating		
II	____	8.	Serves on nursing and/or hospital committees AS ASSIGNED.
	____	9.	Updates clinical practice in accordance with current trends in nursing.

(÷ by 9)

Level	Rating		
III	____	10.	Promotes advancement through the RN Career Ladder.
	____	11.	Communicates current trends and issues in nursing practice to quad/unit staff.
	____	12.	Seeks advanced learning experiences.

(÷ by 12)

Comments (Professional Growth)

APPRAISAL PROFILE:

	A. NURSING PROCESS	B. HUMAN RELATIONS	C. QUALITY ASSURANCE	D. LEADERSHIP/ DECISION-MAKING	E. TEACHING/ DISCHARGE-PLANNING	F. PROFESSIONAL GROWTH	OTHER	ATTENDANCE
4								
3								
2								
1								

Working with the employee, describe GOALS TO BE ACHIEVED BY THE NEXT REVIEW PERIOD.

_____

_____

_____

_____

_____

_____

_____

_____

- EMPLOYEE COMMENTS   (Do you feel your appraisal was accurate?)

_____

_____

_____

_____

_____
Employee Signature/Date

- ABSENT/ILL RECORD   (For Appraisal Period).   .   TARDINESS

- PERSONNEL DEPARTMENT INFORMATION

Current Rate_____   New Rate_____   Effective Date_____

_____ Grant Merit Increase   _____ Consider for Transfer, Termination, Demotion

_____ Withhold Increase Until _____

_____
Rater's Signature/Date

	PM/N

Rater's Immediate Supervisor   Department Head Signature/Date
Signature/Date

Sharon General Hospital

Sharon, Pa.

267 Beds

Behaviorial Performance Assessment: Director, Home Health Agency
Performance Appraisal: R.N. in Emergency Room

Reprinted by permission of Louise C. Hess, R.N., Vice President, Patient
Services; Director of Nursing.

Sharon General Hospital
Sharon, Pennsylvania

BEHAVIORAL PERFORMANCE ASSESSMENT OF DIRECTOR, HOME HEALTH AGENCY

Director, Home Health Agency: _____

Date: _____

Vice President For Patient Services: _____

Directions:

To assess the Director, Home Health Agency

1. Consider performance within the last year.
2. Read each behavior and check either yes or no. Both refer to consistent behavior, i.e., not a one-time error or failure and not a once-only demonstration of the behavior.
3. Identify priority behaviors by placing an asterisk (*) next to the behavior. Priority behaviors are those that should be considered MINIMAL ACCEPTABLE PERFORMANCE for a Director, Home Health Agency. In other words, these would be the priorities of the job or the behaviors so critical to the position that if the Director failed in consistently performing them, she would not be doing her job.

DIRECTOR, HOME HEALTH AGENCY

Responsibilities to Vice President For Patient Services	YES	NO
1. Develops, with staff, yearly measurable objectives.	____	____
2. Directs maintenance of records and reports and submits written communications (memos, reports, etc.) that:		
a) clearly state purpose	____	____
b) are comprehensive and concise	____	____
c) are on appropriate stationery	____	____
3. Demonstrates application of the problem-solving process in all problems reported.	____	____
4. Apprises Vice President For Patient Services of all matters which may require administrative attention.	____	____
Distinguishes between matters requiring prompt attention and those that can wait.	____	____
5. Keeps Vice President For Patient Services aware of necessary interactions with nursing department.	____	____

	YES	NO
6. Makes clinical/administrative decisions that are:		
a) consistent with authority	____	____
b) based on logic	____	____
c) effective	____	____
7. Follows established lines of authority/communication	____	____
8. Communicates and interprets the policies of the Home Health Agency to staff, hospital personnel, physicians and interested others.	____	____
9. Requires staff members to comply with policy.	____	____
10. Effectively resolves conflicts with		
a) employees	____	____
b) physicians	____	____
c) families	____	____
d) other departments.	____	____
11. Delegates responsibility/authority appropriately	____	____
12. Submits an annual budget including capital and personnel requested and justification for either/both.	____	____
13. Initiates methods of cost containment	____	____
14. Staffs agency to meet patient care needs effectively and		
a) comply with agency guidelines	____	____
b) avoid overtime.	____	____
15. Assumes responsibility for Quality Assurance Activities within her department.	____	____
16. Evaluates agency services in relation to audit criteria	____	____
17. Interviews for open positions and discusses with Vice President For Patient Services.	____	____
18. Uses an interpersonal style which can be adjusted to accomplish (with peers, superiors and subordinates) mutually established goals (performance, organizations)	____	____
19. Assists in assuring the quality of care delivered by other members of the health team by the identification and reporting of problems.	____	____
20. Participates in Advisory Committee meetings and furnishes Advisory Committee with pertinent information.	____	____
21. Prepares an annual departmental report.	____	____

Responsibilities to Staff:

	YES	NO
1. Consults with staff to identify, intervene in, and evaluate nursing care on complex/problem patients.	____	____

	YES	NO
2. Communicates the role/function of the Director, Home Health Agency to each member of her staff so that she is utilized as a resource when appropriate.	___	___
3. Ensures that the following regular meetings occur at the agency:		
a) patient care conference	___	___
b) informational staff meetings	___	___
c) staff development sessions.	___	___
4. Provides opportunities for staff to express ideas, offer suggestions and develop plans for implementation	___	___
5. Holds employees accountable for achieving agency objectives.	___	___
6. Monitors staff attendance/punctuality by:		
a) implementing the system for documenting both	___	___
b) reviewing documentation on a regular basis.	___	___
7. Sets goals with employees for improving performance	___	___
8. Gives employees feedback and positive reinforcement on performance.	___	___
9. Evaluates employees objectively and reliably.	___	___
10. Implements the disciplinary action procedure when required.	___	___
11. Ensures that all new employees receive a competency-based, individualized orientation to the agency and position.	___	___
12. Assists staff in collaborating with other health team professionals	___	___
13. Collaborates with Staff Development Department to provide Inservice and Staff Development.	___	___

Responsibilities to Other Health Team Members, Patients and Families.:

	YES	NO
1. Collaborates with other health care professionals for the benefit of patient care.	___	___
2. Solves intra- and interdepartmental, patient/staff, etc., problems when the use of supervisory authority will accomplish the goal.	___	___
3. Contributes to the hospital's operation by participating in committees.	___	___
4. Collaborates with faculty, nursing students, and others to coordinate learning experiences.	___	___
5. Serves as a liaison between Home Health Agency and other community agencies.	___	___

	YES	*NO*
Personal Responsibilities:		

1. Begins work promptly and adheres to days scheduled.   _____   _____
2. Plans work schedule according to the needs of the unit.   _____   _____
3. Submits time schedule to Nursing Office in advance according to Staffing Standards.   _____   _____
4. Demonstrates responsibility for professional growth by:
   a) attending and evaluating in writing continuing education offerings.   _____   _____
   b) suggesting strategies for change   _____   _____
   c) introducing and evaluating changes in agency or administrative activities.   _____   _____

SUMMARY:

RECOMMENDATIONS:

DIRECTOR, HOME HEALTH AGENCY OBJECTIVES:

SIGNATURE_____

DATE_____

VICE PRESIDENT FOR PATIENT SERVICES_____

DATE_____

8/82 JR

Sharon General Hospital
Sharon, Pennsylvania
Nursing Department

Performance Appraisal—Registered Nurse in Emergency Room

NAME _____ UNIT _____ DATE _____ IMMEDIATE SUPERVISOR _____ EVALUATION PERIOD _____

EXPECTED BEHAVIOR

	Y	NI	N

A. IMPLEMENTATION OF THE NURSING PROCESS

1. Completes a nursing assessment on each Emergency Room patient
2. Identifies patient needs based on obtained subjective and objective data
3. Implements appropriate nursing actions to each patient need identified
4. Makes decisions that reflect both knowledge of facts and sound judgment
5. Informs patient and/or significant other about care to be administered
6. Uses self therapeutically in relationships with patients and significant others
7. Records and reports observed physical and emotional reactions to illness, treatment and medications
8. Charts precise and specific observations
9. Identifies and appropriately utilizes health care resource persons to facilitate delivery of nursing care

1. ___ 2. ___ 3. ___ 4. ___ 5. ___ 6. ___ 7. ___ 8. ___ 9. ___

LEGEND

Y —Yes
NI—Needs Improvement
N —No

EXPECTED BEHAVIOR

	Y	NI	N
10. Delegates responsibility for care based on assessment of priorities of patient care needs and the limitations of available health care personnel			
11. Instructs patients in follow-up care after treatment			
12. Evaluates the patient's understanding of instructions given			
13. Evaluates effectiveness of nursing care			
14. Gives written instructions and materials to patients and their families			
15. Teaches preventive health measures to patients and their families			
16. Reports appropriate information to law enforcement and community agencies			

COMMENTS: _____

B. TECHNICAL COMPETENCE

	Y	NI	N
1. Performs procedures and techniques correctly			
2. Maintains asepsis with procedures			
3. Uses equipment according to directives, literature, and operating instructions			
4. Seeks assistance with unfamiliar procedures or situations			
5. Follows established procedure for safe administration of medication and parenteral fluids			
6. Demonstrates knowledge of the nature, purposes and effects of medications			
7. Knows current conditions and status of care for each emergency room patient			
8. Recognizes hazards to patient safety and takes appropriate action to maintain a safe environment and to give patients a feeling of being safe			
9. Responds appropriately to emergency situations			

COMMENTS: _____

EXPECTED BEHAVIOR

	Y	NI	N

C. RELIABILITY

1. Reports on time for duty on all assigned days   1. ___
2. Completes assignment within time schedule   2. ___
3. Complies with policies established for: 3. ___
    a. meal periods   a. ___
    b. breaks   b. ___
    c. dress   c. ___
4. Follows established lines of authority   4. ___
5. Undertakes additional tasks when her own assignments are completed   5. ___

COMMENTS: _____

D. PERSONAL AND PROFESSIONAL GROWTH

1. Demonstrates knowledge of legal boundaries of nursing   1. ___
2. Participates in patient care conferences   2. ___
3. Accepts responsibility for own action   3. ___
4. Evaluates nursing as it is practiced on her unit and takes action to improve clinical expertise   4. ___
5. Offers constructive suggestions for improvement in care of individual patients and in routines on nursing unit   5. ___
6. Attends CPR inservice once yearly   6. ___
7. Attends staff development activities appropriate to learning needs   7. ___
8. Serves on committees when requested   8. ___
9. Serves as preceptor for new employees when requested   9. ___
10. Seeks knowledge in relation to patient condition, disease entity, or treatment   10. ___

EXPECTED BEHAVIOR

Y   NI   N

11. Implements goals set for improved performance   11. ___

COMMENTS: ___
___
___

NURSE'S COMMENTS: ___
___
___

OBJECTIVES SET MUTUALLY BY NURSE AND EMERGENCY ROOM SUPERVI-
SOR: ___
___
___

R.N. ___
SUPERVISOR ___
DATE ___

5/78   8/82 Revised   Revised: 5/83

Index

Framework for Nursing Management, 133
Functions of management, 12, 105, 106, 129
See also specific functions

G

Ganong, Joan M., 2, 12, 13, 14, 26, 28, 30, 31, 33, 117, 118, 122, 123, 127, 130
Ganong, Warren L., 2, 12, 13, 14, 26, 28, 118, 122, 123, 127, 130
Geographical maldistribution of nurses, 134
Gerlach, M.L., 1, 35, 36
G-GRAM: Newsletter for Nurse Managers and Educators, 26
Gilbert, T., 25
Gilmore, M.A., 124
Goals
  See also Objectives; Purpose
  agreement on, 111
  clarification of, 132
  and criticism, 171
  of ESCAPE, 151, 152
  hospital, 58
  individual, 53
  managers oriented toward, 143
  mutual, 100-102, 172
  nursing, 58, 103-105
  organizational, 129
  student participation in setting of, 172
  work unit, 7
Gordon, T., 108
Gosnell, D., 93
Government regulations, 10
  of contracts, 10
  on employment selection procedures, 1
  on performance appraisals, 23
Grade contracting, 157, 158, 172
Griggs v. Duke Power, 36
Grimaldi, P.L., 12, 18
Grop relations skill, 14

Guidelines. *See Uniform Guidelines on Employee Selection Procedures*
Gulack, R., 118

H

Hall, J., 86
Handbook for employees, 60
Hanson, R.L., 16, 17
Harmin, M., 151
Hart, 157
Harvey, A., 155
Head nurse, 222-235
  performance description for, 176-182
Health care concepts, 51-54
HELP with Annual Budgetary Planning, 26
Hierarchy of needs, 6
Historical overview, 1-3
  of career ladders, 118-124
Holistic care, 53
Holley, W.H., 39
Home health agency director, 340-344
Hospital
  budgets of, 58
  goals and objectives of, 58
  organization chart of, 54
  policy manual of, 57
Hospital Research and Educational Trust, 124
House, J., 31
Houston, G., 124
Huey, F., 135, 136
Humanistic psychology, 5
Human needs satisfaction, 6
Human resources planning, 3

I

Incentive programs, 46
Indiana University Hospital, 121
Individual relations of skills, 14
Individuals
  differences in, 6

About the Authors

Joan and Warren Ganong have been a husband-and-wife consulting/writing team for many years. Joan Mary Ganong, R.N., Ph.D., C.M.C. is president of W.L. Ganong Company, Healthcare Management Consultants. She holds a Ph.D. in psychology from The Fielding Institute, Santa Barbara, Calif.; a Master's in nursing; and is the first nurse consultant to become a Certified Management Consultant (C.M.C.).

Warren Lincoln Ganong holds a B.S. degree in industrial engineering from Northeastern University, Boston, and is president emeritus of the W.L. Ganong Company. He is a long-time C.M.C. with broad experience in general industry and healthcare.

In their writings, the Ganongs draw upon their combined expertise in nursing practice, nursing education, and business and industry.

Their other Aspen publications are *Nursing Management* (2nd ed., 1980) and *Cases in Nursing Management* (1979). In addition they are authors and publishers of the *HELP Series of Nursing Management Guides*.

DATE DUE